WALL PILATES WORKOUTS FOR WOMEN

THE COMPLETE ILLUSTRATED STEP-BY-STEP 28-DAY CHALLENGE GUIDE FOR BEGINNERS & SENIORS.

FITNESS PLANNER TO ACHIEVE FLEXIBILITY, STRENGTH, BALANCE, AND LOSE WEIGHT.

BY

Hashtag genYZ

© Copyright 2025. All Rights Reserved.

The publication is sold with the idea that the publisher is not required to render accounting, officially permittedor otherwise qualified services. This document is geared towards providing exact andreliable information concerning the topic and issue covered. If advice is necessary, legal or professional, a practiced individual in the profession should be ordered.

- From a Declaration of Principles which was accepted and approved equally by a Committee of the American Bar Association and a Committee of Publishers and Associations.

In no way is it legal to reproduce, duplicate, or transmit any part of this document in either electronic means or printed format. Recording of this publication is strictly prohibited, and any storage of this document is not allowed unless with written permission from the publisher—all rights reserved.

The information provided here in is stated to be truthful and consistent. Any liability, in terms of inattention or otherwise, by any usage or abuse of any policies, processes, or directions contained within is the sole and utter responsibility of the recipient reader. Under no circumstances will any legal responsibility or blame be held against the publisher for any reparation, damages, or monetary loss due to the information here in, either directly or indirectly.

Respective authors own all copyrights not held by the publisher.

The information here in is offered for informational purposes solely and is universal as so. The presentation of the information is without a contract or any guarantee assurance.

The trademarks that areuse dare without any consent, and the publication of the trademark is without permission or backing by the trademark owner. All trademarks and brands within this book are for clarifying purposes only and are owned by the owners themselves, not affiliated with this document.

TABLE OF CONTENTS

INTRODUCTION 6

CHAPTER 1 10

BEFORE YOU START 10

    LIST OF ALL YOU NEED 11

    YOUR MINDSET 14

    PRECAUTION AND SAFETY TIPS 17

CHAPTER 2: BEGINNER EXERCISE 18

    WALL CHEST STRETCH 19

    WALL CALF STRETCH 20

    WALL SPINE TWIST 21

    SIDE BEND 22

    WALL ANGEL ARMS 23

    WALL ROLL DOWN 25

    RECLINED WALL LEG STRETCH 27

CHAPTER 3 28

INTERMEDIATE EXERCISE 28

    WALL TEASER PREP 29

    WALL ROTATION 30

    WALL DOWN DOG 31

    WALL SQUATS 32

    WALL LUNGE 33

    WALL SIDE LUNGE 34

    WALL BRIDGE 35

    WALL QUAD STRETCH 36

    PUPPY STRETCH 37

    SUPINE WALL TOE TAPS 38

    STANDING SIDE LEG RAISE 39

    WALL SITS WITH ONE LEG EXTENDED 41

    SUPINE WINDSHIELD WIPERS 42

    HIP OPENER 43

    WALL BUTTERFLY 44

    GLUTE BRIDGE WITH KNEE TUCKS 45

- GLUTE BRIDGE WALKS 47
- MARCHING GLUTE BRIDGES 48
- ALTERNATE DONKEY KICKBACKS 49
- REACH THROUGH CRUNCH 50

CHAPTER 4 51

ADVANCE EXERCISE 51
- WALL PLANK 52
- WALL PUSHUP 53
- WALL PIKE 55
- WALL ABDOMINAL CURL 56
- SINGLE-LEG WALL BRIDGE 57

CHAPTER 5 58

28-DAY WALL PILATES EXERCISE CHART 58

WEEK 1: FOUNDATION BUILDING 60
- GENTLE WALL PILATES WARM-UP 61
- WALL SQUATS AND LEG LIFTS 64
- WALL SQUATS WITH ARM RAISES 65
- WALL BRIDGE EXERCISE 66
- WALL PLANKS FOR CORE STRENGTH 67
- WALL 100S 71

WEEK 2: INTERMEDIATE WALL PILATES MOVES 72
- SIDE LEG RAISES ON THE WALL 72
- WALL PILATES PUSHUPS 72

WEEK 3: ADVANCED WALL PILATES CHALLENGE 73
- WALL PIKE EXERCISE 73
- WALL PILATES ROLL-UP 74
- COMBINING MOVES FOR FULL-BODY ENGAGEMENT 77

WEEK 4: MASTERING WALL PILATES FLOW 82
- DYNAMIC WALL PILATES ROUTINE 83
- INCORPORATING PROPS FOR INTENSITY 86
- COOL DOWN AND STRETCHING ON THE WALL 89

CHAPTER 6 90
MINDFULNESS AND BREATHING METHOD FOR WALL PILATES. 90
    BENEFITS OF PROPER BREATHING 91
BONUS CHAPTER.. 93
FITNESS PLANNER FOR SUCCESS 93
    SETTING REALISTIC WALL PILATES GOALS.. 94
    USING THE FITNESS PLANNER EFFECTIVELY 96
    NUTRITION TIPS FOR WALL PILATES SUCCESS 101
CONCLUSION.. 106

INTRODUCTION

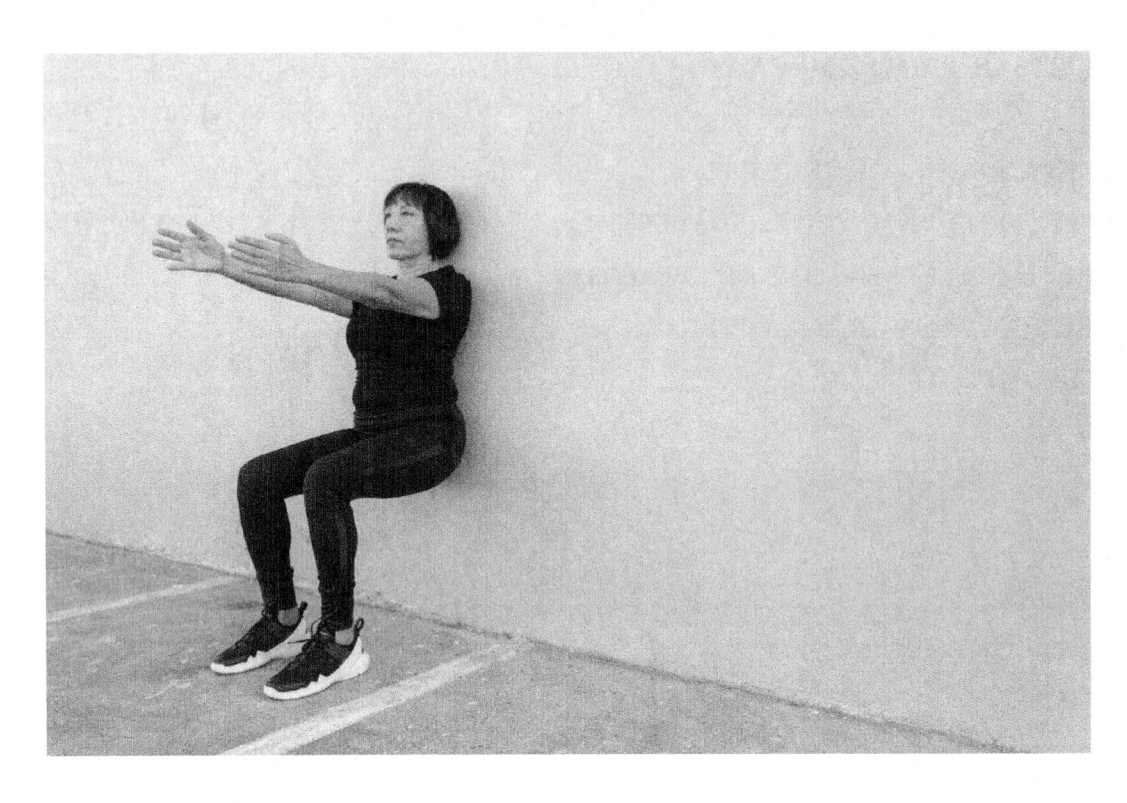

Most women, especially seniors, find it difficult to choose the right exercise to help them stay fit. Going to the gym and buying expensive equipment for the workout is a big turnoff for them due to their age. As such, they prefer a less expensive and easy exercise that would help them achieve the same results as going to the gym and staying fit.

Wall Pilates is best known for its accessibility. This workout can be modified for any fitness level and doesn't require much space or equipment, making it an excellent home workout. In our post-COVID world, everything must be more accessible; gyms closed down in 2020, and more people installed gym equipment at their homes than ever before, leading to at-home workouts becoming ever more popular - following along on a workout video fits well into anyone's schedule - whether working from home or trying to squeeze one in between kids' play.

Wall Pilates is the newest workout trend, delivering impressive results. It is a popular beginner-friendly, low-impact workout focusing on strengthening and toning core muscles. In this version of the traditional Pilates exercise, you push the wall (with your arms, feet, back, or even side) to perform exercises like squats and planks. Using the wall and your body weight, wall Pilates works for various muscle groups and intensifies specific exercises.

Pilates originated in New York City in the post-WWI era. Invented by Joe and Clara Pilates, the method began when Joe served as an orderly in a hospital in Germany, helping veterans who were unable to walk. He rigged parts of beds to help support the patients' limbs as they worked through the method. After immigrating to the US, he opened his first studio in New York City and published a booklet called "Your Health" and "The Return to Life through Contrology," which he practiced throughout his life. Pilates was only applied to the method after Joe died in 1967.

Pilates was based on three principles – Breath, Whole-body Health, and Whole-body Commitment. The core foundation of Pilates includes breath, concentration, centering, control, precision, and flow. Clara Pilates shared this method with apprentices in her first studio, and it continues to be practiced today. The popularity of Pilates has grown, with countless studios popping up worldwide.

Wall Pilates is essentially the same workout Joe and Clara Pilates shared nearly 80 years ago in New York City. It enlists using a wall to create resistance and help develop more strength. The wall mimics the foot bar used in formal Pilates exercises. Since no equipment is needed (only a wall), anyone can complete a Wall Pilates workout at home, in a hotel, or anywhere with a wall.

One of the main reasons people first turn to Pilates is due to health-related concerns like osteoporosis or arthritis. Furthermore, this exercise poses no significant injury risk.

Wall Pilates is an exceptional way to stretch and realign the spine, creating better alignment for optimal spine health. This exercise also emphasizes core muscles like abs, glutes, and back muscles, which improve core strength by helping reduce unhealthy curvatures of the spine - ultimately leading to improved posture while strengthening core muscles, resulting in spinal alignment that relieves backache or stiffness.

Wall Pilates is perfect for managing chronic back pain or simply becoming more active and healthier through gentle moves that focus on strengthening core muscle groups and providing balance, flexibility, and alignment.

Wall Pilates' greatest advantage lies in not requiring expensive equipment like a Reformer, Wunda Chair, or any heavy items to derive its many benefits. Simply using a mat and nearby wall as support and immediate feedback compared to practicing on a mat can bring immediate feedback; some seemingly easy exercises may become more challenging due to being upright; furthermore, its support provides back, hip, and shoulder relief; making this workout suitable even when space or equipment constraints limit workout options at home or while traveling; therefore making Wall Pilates ideal - even preferable over studio workouts!

Wall Pilates is particularly helpful to women as an exercise to improve posture, balance, and flexibility. Furthermore, this form of fitness provides a fantastic mind-body connection by strengthening kinesthesia (where one's body exists in space). With regular Wall Pilates practice, you will also increase mobility by increasing your motion range - helping to bring awareness of self to every exercise routine you undertake. Being mindful during exercise sessions will bring greater understanding to body awareness.

Pilates has proven its worth to many athletes for its ability to strengthen coordination and build strength. Wall Pilates will make you strong, stretched, and more accurate, and perform balanced movements in whatever sport it may be used in.

Expectant mothers can benefit immensely from wall Pilates during pregnancy as it offers an adaptable form of exercise to accommodate all stages of their gestation and get the body ready for work. By pairing breathing exercises with Wall Pilates exercises, stress will be eased away while relaxing the body and mind. Wall Pilates' adaptable form can easily fit your pregnancy journey; its intensity can adjust according to your best suit.

Wall Pilates also helps in easing menstrual cramps by stretching and opening your pelvis and the muscles on your lower back to alleviate any associated discomfort. Enhancing circulation to your pelvic floor may reduce inflammation, making a stronger pelvic floor even more effective at controlling bladder control and increasing sexual satisfaction!

Wall Pilates and general Pilates workouts can help enhance both the quantity and quality of sleep by relieving stress and practicing deep breathing techniques.

Wall Pilates can be an excellent exercise option for injured, pregnant, and older individuals who struggle to get off the floor, as it eliminates harder moves. Furthermore, this form of physical therapy offers relief if lying flat on your back is physically impossible or impractical for extended periods and provides opportunities to strengthen posture, balance, and alignment while increasing fitness and well-being.

This exercise can add variety and variety to your Pilates practice or routine. Being portable and convenient, this workout can even be completed during travel or work breaks - it even utilizes walls as additional props, providing another challenge to strengthen upper body strength and mobility.

Pilates might be the most efficient form of exercise for helping with weight loss; it burns fewer calories than running or cycling.

However, Pilates shouldn't be disregarded; rather, it can help increase your likelihood of maintaining a healthy weight over time by helping control emotional eating and strengthening muscle tone for easier physical activity.

Wall Pilates has turned out to be popular, prompting social media users to organize month-long wall Pilates challenges and post-before-and-after photos of those participating - some as popular as Rachel's Fit Pilates Challenge with nearly one million YouTube views! The results can be truly remarkable!

Renee Mowatt noticed changes to her body after just one month of practicing wall Pilates four to five times weekly for four months on TikTok -- now with over 12 million views -- which she discovered. Renee found exceptional results from this workout and now shares it with others wanting to try it.

Applying wall Pilates into your routine can help target areas like the belly, arms, abs, and core strength. Wall Pilates exercises utilize a wall as additional support and resistance, making them accessible even to beginners looking to tone specific parts of their bodies or shed belly fat.

Wall Pilates exercises provide a convenient way of working out daily and suit different fitness levels. Arm routines, targeted ab workouts, and plank variations are available on these workouts.

This Wall Pilates Workouts Book will open up a world of fitness discoveries! Packed with clear instructions and illustrations in every chapter, mindfulness techniques will simultaneously teach how to elevate the body and mind. Starting the wall Pilates journey has never been simpler! This book also ensures it remains safe for seniors.

With this fully illustrated exercise workout guide, Wall Pilates is accessible and achievable from the convenience of your home- helping you achieve full-body fitness, strength, and flexibility. The 28-Day Wall Pilates Challenge Exercise plan has been tailored specifically for every fitness level to make progress an attainable goal.

Let's get started!

CHAPTER 1

BEFORE YOU START

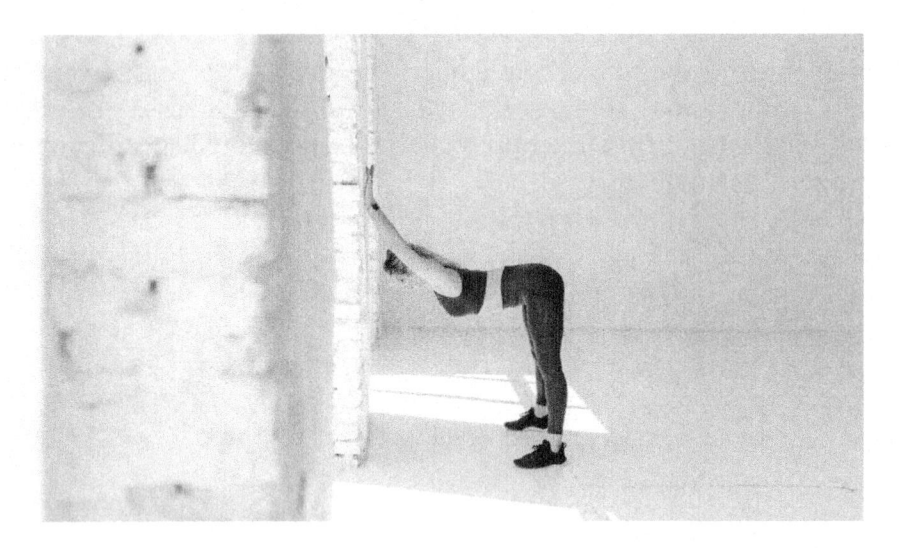

Understanding the basics of Pilates exercise is helpful for anyone interested in wall Pilates, yet its popularity has increased significantly due to its accessibility for beginners. Before beginning wall Pilates for the first time, remember a few things before making your debut session.

Before investing in equipment needed for wall pilates, why should you select this apparatus over traditional solutions?

Wall pilates equipment can be more cost-effective. By mounting directly to walls instead of taking up floor space diagonally across them, these units take up less space on your floor - making them the ideal option for home Pilates practice.

Classic Pilates provides an intensive coreburn, but its workout doesn't offer as much muscle challenge due to the setup of the table. On the contrary, Wall Pilates equipment may present more of a physical challenge, particularly to your lower body muscles.

Three primary wall units are currently available that you may want to consider when choosing your ideal home or studio machine.

A ladder Unit - This device contains wooden planks from top to bottom, enabling users to hang it at different heights for increased workout difficulty levels. Instead of springs, this unit contains elastic bands.

Classic springboard units - featuring wooden backrest panels to add stability for explosive workouts that involve pulling and additional attachments than their ladder-type or minimalistic designs counterparts - have long been considered one of the top fitness tools available.

Minimalistic Design - This design features an open back with wooden platforms on either end that secure walls securely. Depending on their manufacturer, these units may contain as few or as many springs as their wooden counterpart.

LIST OF ALL YOU NEED

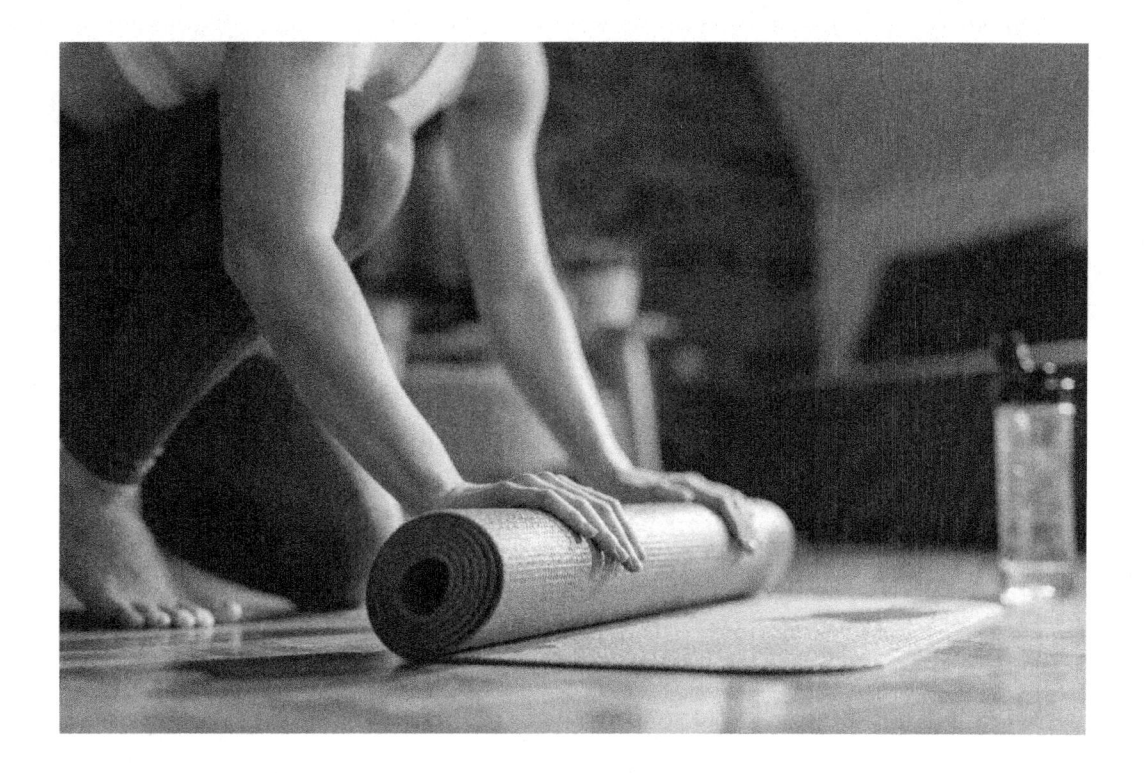

Wall Pilates exercises can be done without equipment, but with a few helpful tools you can maximize, speed up and enhance the beneficial effects of these exercises.

Some recommended tools include:

• A yoga mat: for comfort and cushioning

• Resistance bands: for added challenge and to target specific muscle groups

• Pilates balls: to improve balance and core strength

• Small weights: to increase the intensity of your workout

These tools will help you get the most out of your Wall Pilates practice and reach your fitness goals faster.

Strengthening your core and increasing your body's flexibility at home is easy with the increasing popularity of wall Pilates. People who are ready to start need equipment to enhance their home Pilates routine. If you don't have the money to purchase an expensive wall-mounted unit, doing the fad Wall Pilates at home can be the best alternative. To ensure you make the most of the pilates at home, check out this equipment checklist to start your workout!

A STRONG WALL

The wall must be strong. That is perhaps the primary prerequisite for Pilates on the wall. It should be strong enough to support your body weight when exercising.

MATS

Also, it would help if you chose a high-quality Pilates mat with great cushioning and grip. The mat you choose should be strong in width and long enough to fit the entire physique. It offers soft padding to rest your back against the floor.

RESISTANCE BANDS

Resistance bands are a crucial accessory to the wall Pilates equipment collection, with various types of resistance bands in size and strength to suit any exercise intensity. Choose the right resistance band based on your capabilities and desired workout intensity to tailor your workout. Resistance bands are excellent for building muscle mass and improving resistance training in any exercise, not just Pilates.

PILATES BALL

You'll need a Pilates ball for exercises primarily focusing on balance and core strength. Like resistance bands, ball exercises are more challenging than classic exercises. They're ideal for Pilates workouts that focus on the lower body, core (legs and hips), and glutes) wall planks, pushups, stretching, and extension exercises.

ANKLE-WORTHS

Training for strength using exercise that resistance can build your legs' strength.

THE PILATES RING

This is particularly beneficial for isometric hold and targeted toning.

Foam Rollers are designed to aid in the recovery of muscles and increase flexibility.

PILATES BLOCKS

These blocks assist certain poses that are difficult to perform.

YOUR MINDSET

Many have trouble with Pilates as it's different from others – what may appear to be higher-intensity exercises. Training with weights or running like running, for instance, usually requires you to complete a certain distance or reps. Pilates, meanwhile, requires focus and control. You are forced to slow down and have fewer distractions, and it's extremely difficult.

Incredibly, even as you gain strength, Pilates never gets easier as you continue to practice you do; the better your posture improves and, consequently, the more challenging it is to feel. Don't let this hinder you from doing your best. The more difficult it is, the more efficient it will be.

Although this equipment for wall Pilates can help you in your workout, it is not required. The most important thing is your dedication to regular exercise and balancing difficult workouts with adequate relaxation. Enroll your mat, gear up, and prepare to see your body transform one step at a time!

Here are some tips to improve your attitude toward a wall pilates workout

IT'S A JOURNEY

The pop culture that makes you believe that Pilates might be the best option for getting six-pack abs and a look that resembles models like the Victoria's Secret model. However, it's more about being part of a continuous journey rather than not achieving the goal.

The results you see (toning muscles, a better posture, and flexibility) can be gradual, so it's important to take your time and concentrate on the process, not the final desired result.

If you're starting and haven't been working out or pilates regularly, adding wall workouts into your exercise routine can be beneficial since you'll be burning more calories than before. Reducing calories is a key component of the body's composition.

Suppose you are new to Pilates. In that case, wall Pilates can assist you in getting familiar with the practice as it helps stabilize alignment and modify exercises.

If you know your Pilates training is possible, Wall Pilates can provide some challenges. However, it's not the only choice in Pilates.

If you want to change your body's shape, I suggest an intense form of Pilates, such as dynamic Pilates, and adding additional resistance using resistance bands and weights to make things more challenging. As with everything else, it is important to be consistent and advance your training as you get stronger to give your body new obstacles continuously.

Also, be aware that a transformation in body composition can be multifaceted. The results can be affected by hormones, sleep quality, the genetics of stress, the level of activity and diet, and a calorie deficiency.

START SLOW

There's no set rule. However, most experts suggest exercising Pilates at least three times a week. This allows your body time to recuperate between exercises. Slowing down and not pushing yourself too hard when you're beginning is best. Once you're at ease with your workouts, you can increase the frequency and intensity of your exercise routines.

As you begin, certain moves may appear impossible. Moving your legs and arms is a common mistake. It provides you with momentum, meaning that your muscles aren't able to pull their weight. Begin with small steps and gradually increase the number of movements. As your strength and flexibility improve, you'll be able to achieve more.

The longer you wait between each workout, the more time your muscles are tense, making them feel more invigorated. Indeed, research from the Journal of Physiology showed that an increase in Time Under Tension (TUT) could make exercises more difficult and increase the growth of muscles. Another study revealed that slowing down exercises can make them more difficult since they require coordination, stability, balance, agility, power, and strength.

BREATHWORK

Breathwork is among Joseph Pilates' key principles. It requires the engagement of your core's transverse and deep abdominal muscles. For instance, this might be the occasion to slow down and relax while lifting weights.

Breathwork is a key component of Pilates. Training programs that focus on breathing deeply and evenly assist in bringing oxygen to muscles while relaxing the whole body.

If you gasp for air while doing Pilates exercises, your technique might need adjustment. Stop and focus on your breathing before continuing the exercise. Deep breathing has immense benefits over and above Pilates and can help lower stress levels and improve overall health.

CORE ENGAGEMENT

Engaging your core is essential to each Pilates exercise. The core is comprised of your back, abdominal, and hip muscles. Engaging them is vital to protecting your lower back and making your exercises more efficient. Although working your core and its various parts might initially seem overwhelming, try focusing on working just one part simultaneously until they all work in harmony!

Through practice, you'll soon be able to focus your body without thinking. One way to determine whether you're engaged correctly is to see if your stomach cramps when breathing in. If you notice this, then you're doing the right thing!

MODIFYING THE EXERCISE YOU USE

There's no reason to be ashamed of making adjustments to make exercises easier or more difficult. It's a good idea to encourage this as your endurance and flexibility grow as time passes. The sooner you can do this, the better. You've started these new challenges; do it.

If you find an exercise too difficult to handle, do not be scared of trying to complete it and doing another easier version. It's important to find something that is challenging but doesn't become excessive.

ASK ATTENTION TO YOUR BODY

Pilates can be considered an exercise with low impact; however, that doesn't mean it is safe. Be aware of the body's signals and try not to push too hard. You should stop the exercise if you feel discomfort or pain. Take plenty of water and warm up before performing all Pilates exercises.

Technique and time under tension complexity are two of the most important aspects of Pilates' progress. It isn't always easy to keep track of progress when doing Pilates. Lifting weights is simpler as you lift a higher weight or perform more repetitions.

It is possible to utilize the time in tension as a progress factor, but it's not simple to monitor. It will require you to stop after each exercise to track how long you were doing it. Determining the muscles used and the length of time is nearly impossible. Therefore, shape is the best measurement to keep track of.

Running, for example, can be able to see your speed increasing, and with weights, you will see your body getting stronger.

GET HELP

Asking for help from a qualified Pilates teacher is a great idea for anyone new to Pilates. They will teach you the proper technique for each exercise and help you perform exercises safely. If you cannot pay for private lessons, various internet-based resources (books, videos, etc.) can help you get started.

Remember these before you begin your Pilates journey so you'll soon be on the way to a healthier, stronger body within minutes.

The drawback of wall Pilates, as with the other Pilates performed at home alone, is that you do not receive any feedback or instruction from a professional instructor. Practicing the right position, performing your movements precisely, applying your breath properly, and using the right muscles to reap maximum advantages are essential. You may require some assistance if you're new to yoga and need help.

Sometimes (especially when doing intensive exercises), you could do worse harm than benefit when you're not correctly engaging your core. However, this rarely happens; I believe it's better than bad.

Wall Pilates can be restrictive and boring if it's your only exercise. I love using equipment like props or weights to create additional challenges and obstacles. Therefore, I recommend changing your workout routine by using your floor to perform plank exercises where you utilize your body weight to create impossible resistance against walls.

PRECAUTION AND SAFETY TIPS

Pilates is a wonderful complement to other forms of exercise. Strengthening your core can make other events, such as running, easier and less likely to cause injury. As with any exercise regimen, listening to your body and avoiding overexertion is important. Consult your healthcare provider before starting wall Pilates if you have any existing medical conditions. Start with beginner-friendly exercises and progress gradually.

When diving into your home wall Pilates workouts, ensure your space is optimized for safety and effectiveness. Begin by clearing the area surrounding your wall Pilates unit of any sharp or hard objects. This precaution significantly reduces the likelihood of injury if you lose balance during exercise. Furthermore, always remember to warm up before starting your routine. Warming up conditions your body for the exercises ahead and minimizes the risk of strained or pulled muscles.

Muscle soreness after Pilates is normal and typically subsides after one or two days of practice.

If the soreness lasts longer than a few days or is accompanied by swelling, redness, or fever, seek medical advice immediately. Overuse could injure muscles or joints, and they will provide personalized advice on recovering.

Wall Pilates can be done safely under proper guidance and supervision, providing gentle exercise that engages deliberate motions, activates core muscles, and utilizes walls as resistance and support - helping build stronger muscles while increasing flexibility. But as with any exercise regimen, it must be approached logically for maximum results.

Wall Pilates' success requires learning the appropriate techniques from a certified instructor, tailoring exercises to your fitness level, and paying attention to any discomfort caused by using stable equipment.

Consider taking extra steps to enhance your workout practices. Purchase a quality mat, which will provide necessary support during floor exercises and make clean-up much simpler; wear comfortable clothing (no loose-fitting garments that might get caught in equipment or limit movements); invest in non-slip socks, which offer greater grip; and pause or stop your session when feeling tired to rest and recover before continuing with your session.

Before engaging in Wall Pilates, individuals with preexisting health concerns should consult their healthcare provider to ensure it fits their physical condition and capabilities - as with any new fitness regime.

By following these safety guidelines and tips, your wall Pilates workouts can become both rejuvenating and enjoyable components of your daily routine.

CHAPTER 2: BEGINNER EXERCISE

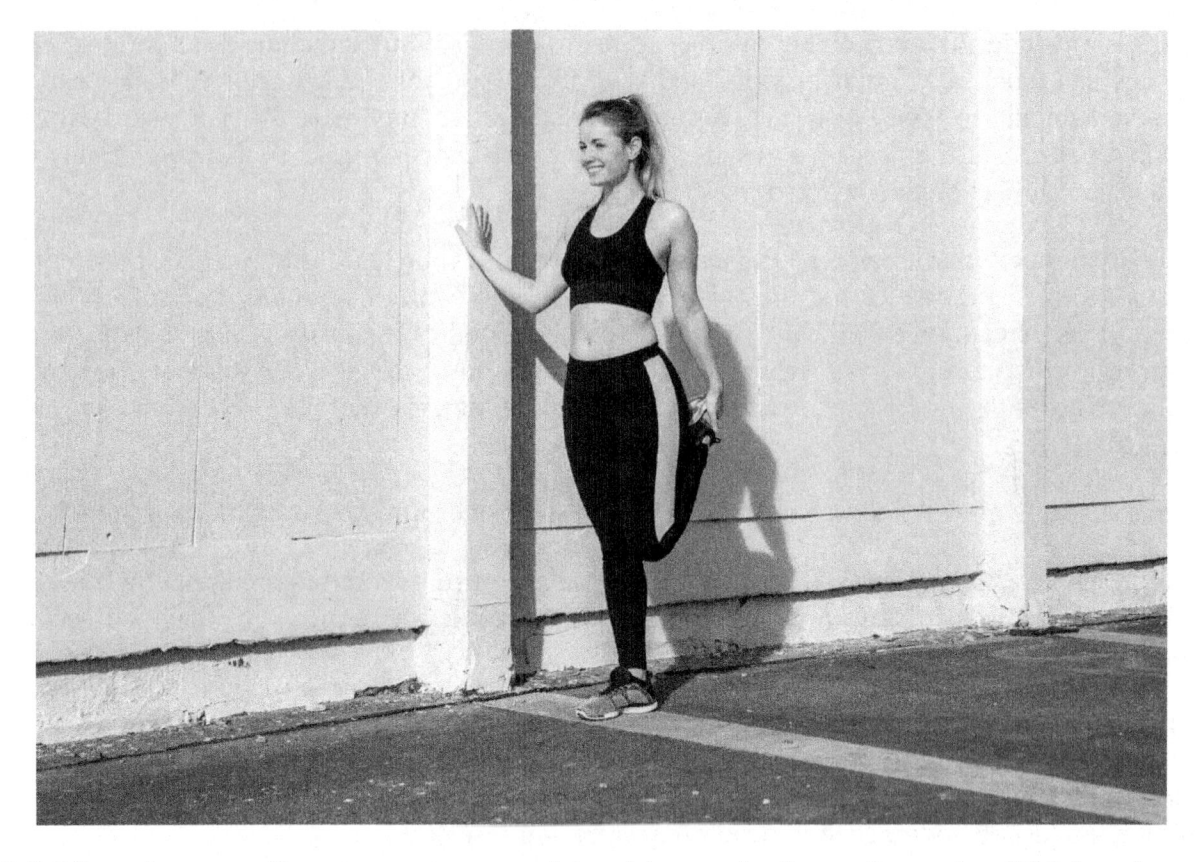

Wall Pilates is an excellent way to start practicing this popular form of exercise. With low-impact and gentle exercises such as the hundred, wall Pilates provides an ideal, supportive environment where beginners can build their confidence as they advance.

Here at Pure Pilates, we have created one of the top beginner wall Pilates workout routines with simple yet challenging exercises designed for beginner wall Pilates routines, providing an all-over strengthening Pilates workout.

Below are some top beginner wall Pilates exercises for a full-body Pilates workout!:

WALL CHEST STRETCH

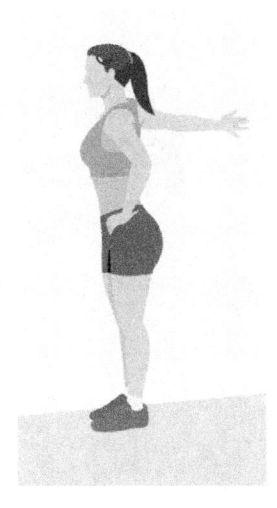

Desk work, driving, swimming, and carrying boxes all utilize arms and chest muscles to perform their tasks. Many of our lives occur in front of us, leading us to use muscles from this area more frequently and often becoming hypertonic (shortened), thus restricting chest and shoulder arm flexibility.

Chest stretches are a good method of increasing the flexibility of the chest muscles and connective tissue and improving the flexibility of shoulders to help improve upper-body posture and pain-free movements.

This exercise allows you to stretch your chest independently.

DIRECTIONS

- To accomplish it, you must take the split stance, with one leg forward and the other the left leg behind - in the wall at the end or in a doorway. Relax your right arm away from your body.
- Lift the left arm to the level of its shoulders and then place it on an exterior wall or entranceway, bent elbow 90 degrees.
- Press your chest gently through wide space until you feel the stretch.
- Moving or lifting an arm can allow you to stretch different chest areas.
- Repeat on the other side.

WALL CALF STRETCH

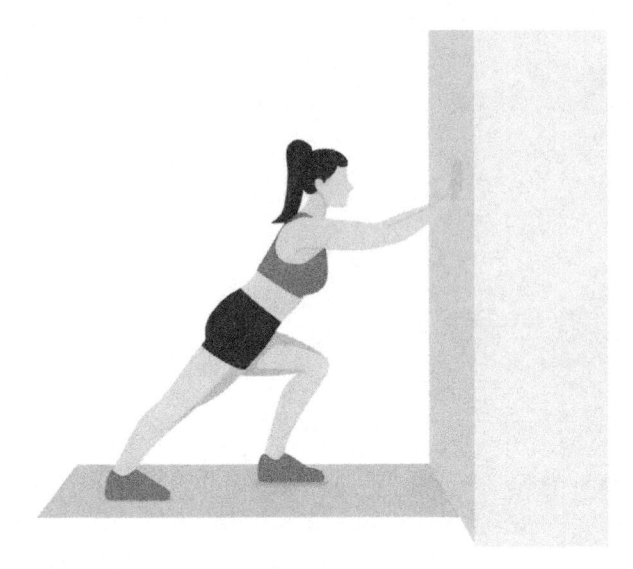

Wall Pilates exercise for beginners is perfect for those who want to master the correct squat posture without causing knee pain. Utilizing an exercise wall, this one helps to ensure the proper alignment of the ankles and knees.

This workout is great for new wall Pilates users since it doesn't require you to be on the ground. Adding the calf raise allows this exercise to work simultaneously for all the important muscle groups in your lower back!

DIRECTIONS

To ensure maximum efficiency and success, be sure to follow these steps:

- Put your back against the wall and then step your feet out slightly while you move your hips and knees 90 degrees until your body is upright.
- Keep your back against the wall while pressing your belly button towards your spine to stimulate your core muscles.
- Make sure your thighs are in line with your floor, parallel to one another, and have knees directly under your knees, placed together and not extended over ankles.
- Arms extend in front of your body so they don't get in the way of your leg muscles.
- After holding the place for five minutes, raise your heels off the ground and then roll your weight on your toes to perform a calf raise. It would help if you remained in a squat posture.
- Then, press through your feet's ball, point your toes forward, and slowly lower your feet. Repeat the process.
- Perform 10 Calf raises while in a Squat Hold position against the Wall.

WALL SPINE TWIST

Perform this relaxing spinal twist with a wall; the back and neck will be grateful for it. Utilizing resistance from walls helps to increase your stretch. It's more effective than doing it on your own. Sitting spine twists are excellent for increasing side-to-side flexibility within the spine. But consider using resistance from a wall to get a more intense twist experience! Try the second variant if the first option isn't enough for you.

DIRECTIONS

- Begin by sitting near the wall. Relax your back and place your legs against the wall with the knees bent. Push your butt against the wall and keep your back up.
- Straighten your feet against a wall while keeping your heels resting on it to begin your Legs Up the Wall pose. Lower both knees, bend them, and lower them to your left side, putting your feet on the wall once more.
- Spread your arms wide into the T-position and look directly toward your eyes.
- When you have taken five deep or longer breaths, raise both knees towards your chest, then roll over onto your right side while looking away for five breaths, while looking leftwards for five breaths.
- Return to Spinal Twist on the left side.
- Stretch your left leg outwards until it rests against the wall, and allow the right leg to drop over it to create a more pronounced spine twist.
- Hold this position for five or more minutes (you might hear a few pops!) before lifting both legs off the ground and repeating the same stretch on the opposite side.

SIDE BEND

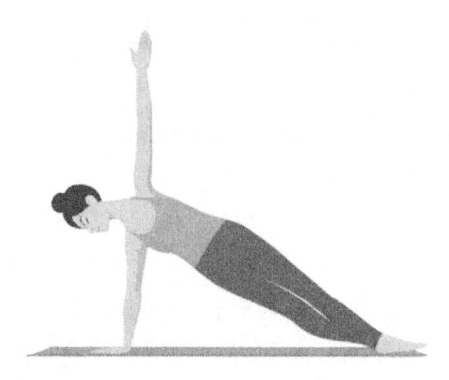

A side bend is a great way to open the side body, including the shoulders and hips. If you like the Side Kicks on the Pilates Mat, you will enjoy the Side Bend. It's another side-body exercise that needs all the strength you learned from your sidekicks.

While this exercise resembles yoga in many ways, be mindful that its focus remains within your seat rather than pushing up onto one shoulder alone. When starting, you could stagger your feet to create more surface area and hold and lower with control until reaching a final lower lift at the end - this may take practice!

DIRECTIONS

To complete it properly, follow these directions:

- Lift and stack your hips while opening your chest, holding for 30 seconds before sitting on one hip with one hand slightly in front of your shoulder with fingers pointed away from you and your hand parallel to your feet.
- Your knees start bent slightly. If you were to look at your hands and feet, they would be in one straight line, while your seat and your knees would be on either side of that line.
- To perform, pull your shoulder back, press your bottom hip up, stand on your hands and feet, lift both hips to an upright position, hold, then carefully lower back down onto the mat - repeat two more times before holding for the final time.
- If this goes smoothly, keep your legs straight while lifting and lowering your hips three times. Your top arm may move up and over before backing down alongside you as you look directly ahead to avoid straining or twisting your neck.
- When finished on one side, return to your starting position and repeat. Immediately swing your legs over to the other side (you could also tease them over to this side) before switching sides again for more repetitions on that side.

Every one of us has a strong side and a weak side. If you find one side is much stronger than the other, do the weak side first, then the strong side, and then the weak side again.

WALL ANGEL ARMS

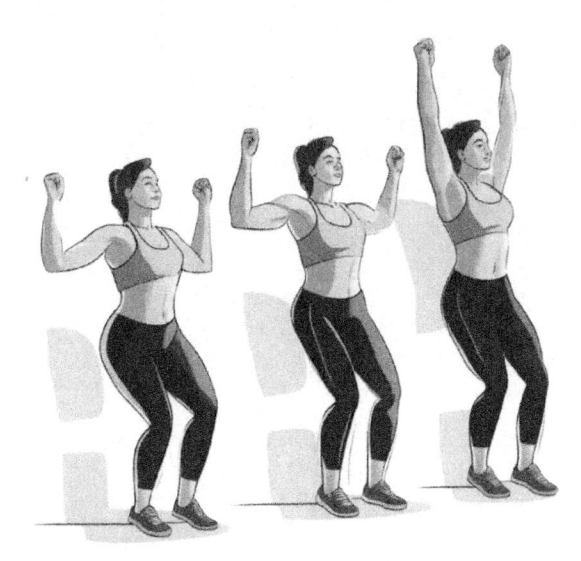

Wall angel is a basic exercise, but it can be very demanding based on where you are in your journey to mobility.

All you require is a place to stand, or you could lie on your floor with your knees bent. To strengthen the muscles in your arms, stand in front of the wall, spread your arms out to the sides, and then rotate your arms around in circles.

This exercise could aid:

- Move the shoulder girdle
- Reduce a head's forward position
- Lift the chest and lower shoulders. This is done by stretching muscles in the back of the body.
- Actively build up the rhomboids and middle and lower traps on the back.
- Lower tension in the traps on top.

DIRECTIONS:

- Place your back against the wall. Place your feet between 6 and 12 inches from the wall, keeping your knees bent slightly.
- Lean your middle back against the wall. Flatten your back to the wall using the posterior pelvic tilt.
- Make sure to tuck your chin a bit, allowing you to increase the length of your neck. Put the side of your head against the wall, keeping the chin tucked.
- Lower your shoulders from your ears.
- The arms should be raised to 90 degrees. And place your elbows on the wall, then place them on your hands on the backs.

- Slowly raise your arms over your head until you are in the Y-shape. While doing this, ensure you are in close contact using your entire head, back, elbows, and hands while keeping your shoulder blades in the downward exercise.
- Make sure that the repetitions are slow and controlled.
- This is a basic but effective workout that you can perform regularly. You can try three times of 10, which you can alternate throughout the day to keep you active and moving.

Modifications

If you feel restricted in your shoulders and can't keep them from the wall, start the exercise by slightly placing your arms and elbows away. You can get the shoulders back, elbows, and hands in the wall when you get stronger.

To make the exercise more difficult, narrow the Y-shape and make your heels closer to the wall while keeping in contact with everything against the wall.

WALL ROLL DOWN

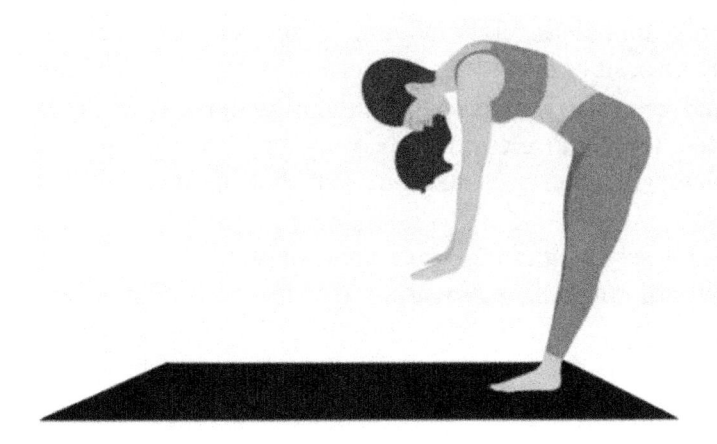

Wall roll-down is an excellent exercise to open the back and hips while engaging the abdominals, like roll-up on a mat. As with roll-up, wall roll-down can help open your body by engaging the abdominals while opening up your back and hips while stretching and engaging hamstrings for stretching back, working abs, and teaching good posture all at the same time.

Wall roll-down is a simple standing mat exercise that engages the abdominals to create the articulated curve of the spine. It is often used in Pilates exercises like roll-ups on the mat. Use your abs to achieve that articulated curve often used by Pilates practitioners! Like its mat counterpart, wall roll-down engages abs to achieve that articulated spine curve Pilates practitioners strive for when practicing Pilates' work! Stretch back and hamstrings while working abdominals, and stretch back and hamstrings while teaching good posture!

This workout is ideal for Pilates novices to get used to strengthening their abdominal muscles and relaxing their shoulders, where most people keep tension. This exercise can be used to relieve stress at any time throughout the day! The tight neck and swollen shoulders of a person with strained shoulder muscles can cause bad posture. Awareness of your body will aid in improving posture by breathing more deeply while improving your walking form and alleviating stress on your back, neck, hips, knees, and legs.

DIRECTIONS:

- Stand high against a wall and rest your body against it while placing your feet between 6 and 10 inches away. Shift your feet six to 10 inches until they are again in contact with it.
- Pull in your abdominals as you keep shoulders away from ears and arms straight at your sides with arms outstretched, making the chest wide while simultaneously dropping ribs down for inhalation/exhalation exercises. Inhale.
- After exhaling, tilt your head as you slowly pull off your back, separating the vertebra from the vertebra. Your abdominals should remain elevated while you feel as if your spine lengthens as you move down. Your arms align with your ears, and your arms are in sync with your body, moving down until parallel to your ears.
- After each session, you can deepen the abs' sculpt and slowly move off the walls while stretching your neck and head muscles.

- As far as you can without letting your hips go off the wall. Inhale as long as you can. Keep your abdominals tight while being aware of your curve in your middle, upper, and lower sections evenly spread throughout your torso's upper middle and lower sections throughout the body - possibly providing the perfect stretch to your hamstrings.
- Begin to exhale and climb to the wall by executing an upward roll with your lower abdominals. Utilizing these muscles to help bring your pelvis up is an effective move. After you've completed the exercise, take one vertebra up at a time, putting each one on the walls as you move.
- When standing upright as you stand up, you should notice a moment when your ribs drop and your shoulders fall into place, creating the feeling of moving your upper body between the shoulders. When this moment is achieved, you should return to your starting position, ensuring your abs are in place and your shoulders have sunk to their proper positions.

Common Errors (indicated below)

Avoid these common mistakes to reap the maximum benefits from this exercise. It will also help prevent stress.

- Speeding Up: For maximum efficiency, you should exercise slowly and vertebra by vertebra under control. Going more quickly will not let you experience the full benefit.
- Shoulders that are raised: Ensure you have shoulders that are at ease. Relax tension. This feeling is crucial to a good posture. Re-examining the posture of Pilates could be helpful.
- Forcing Stretch: Don't force yourself to go further than you are comfortable with. This isn't about reaching for the toe touch but rather rolling as low as possible without letting your hips fall off the wall or straining yourself.

RECLINED WALL LEG STRETCH

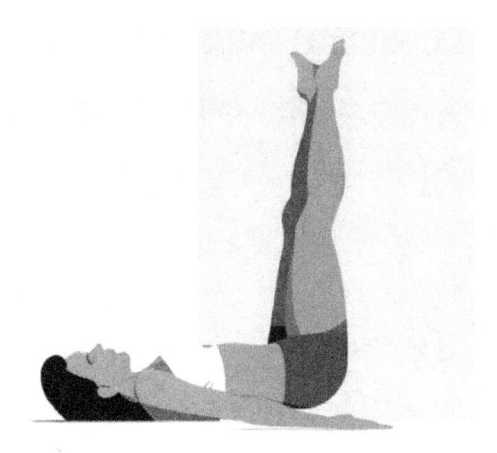

To work your lower abs and core, lie on your back with your legs against the wall and raise and lower them. Avoid inverted poses during menstruation. Use the wall for support if you have low blood pressure. Don't practice on a full stomach.

Benefits

- Soothes tired, stressed legs and feet
- Improves circulation
- Calms the mind
- Reduces anxiety and fatigue
- Therapeutic for headaches and mild depression

DIRECTIONS

- Sit sideways, close to a wall. Your right hip and side body should nearly touch the wall.
- Gently swing your legs up the wall while reclining back onto your forearms or rolling your shoulders under.
- Scoot hips close to the wall. Legs remain relatively straight and hip-width apart.
- Arms can rest on the floor by your sides with palms up.
- Relax your neck and close your eyes. Breathe deeply for 2-5 minutes.
- Bend knees to release. Gently roll to your side before coming up to sit.

CHAPTER 3

INTERMEDIATE EXERCISE

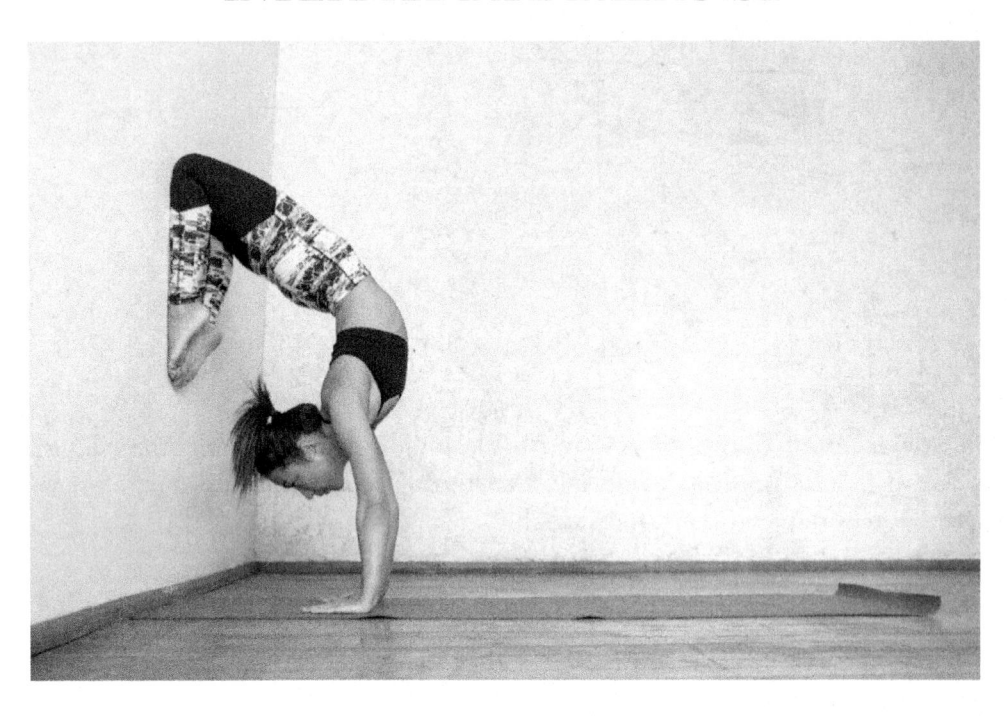

You want to start but aren't sure you're up for an hour-long wall Pilates workout yet. That's okay! You can try these Pilates wall exercise routines at your home to better understand the format for this exercise.

These moves can be taken when you travel. Each hotel room is divided into four walls; they don't fill every square inch of space with furniture.

WALL TEASER PREP

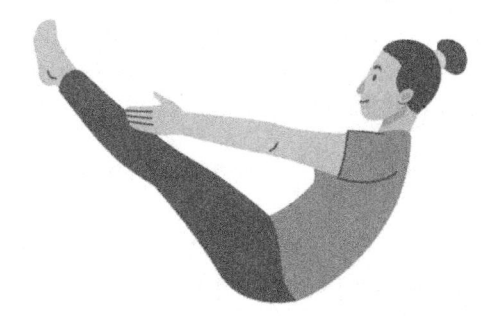

Teaser is not a peak Pilates pose, but it reveals where you need to work more in your Pilates practice. And it's the exercise that hangs everyone up. So many things can be a culprit to you "getting" the Teaser on the Pilates Mat. And you must know that some exercises and preps will help you get to the Teaser when your body is ready for that day. Use this to prepare your Teaser and bring them back out when you need extra support.

Focus on exercises that support the part of the Teaser that is difficult.

As you do these, remember that Teaser is not THE Pilates pose. It's just one of the most recognizable. And, when Teasers are being called out in a class, use these exercises until you are ready to try them.

DIRECTIONS

Rolling like a Ball into Teaser: Sitting in a Rolling Like a ball shape rock back, and then as you come up, straighten your legs and arms and reach for your high diagonal. Bend your knees, roll them back into a ball, and repeat.

Single Leg Teaser: Start seated up, knees bent, feet and knees squeezing together. Stretch one leg out straight, keeping the knees and legs together. It is easier to have your arms hold your legs; harder arms reach for the level of your toes. Roll your upper body down and up 3x and switch.

Half Roll Back: Both knees are bent, and the upper body rolls down and back up.

The more you connect your arms to your back, the easier it is to reach your body up and over with your arms.

WALL ROTATION

The wall can strengthen your abs, lower back and oblique the hamstrings, quads, and glutes for a total training session that improves core strength, tightens and the muscles, improves posture, stability, and postures, and strengthens legs.

DIRECTIONS

- Start this squat workout by placing your legs straight and your back pressed against a wall while holding a medicine ball or dumbbell with both hands.
- Turn your body right before changing directions by turning leftward.
- Repeat until the set is finished.

Proper Breathing Forms and Forms

It's done when your legs are bent at 90 degrees and your ankles are aligned and parallel to the floor. Then, you can twist your torso upwards from your ribcage and breathe out.

Learn to practice wall sits and Russian Twists. Get started with wall sits and Russian twists before moving to wall sitting in a rotation using 30-second to one-minute sessions on the walls. Once comfortable with your technique, move around on the wall for 30-second or 1-minute sets.

WALL DOWN DOG

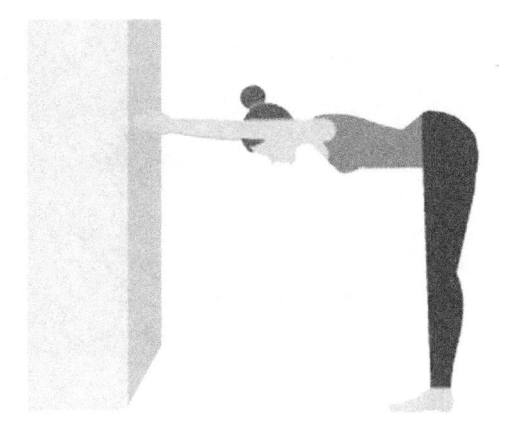

A downward-facing dog at the wall is a great way to practice the pose without the weight of our bodies on the wrists and shoulders. It helps us find the alignment of the wrist, shoulder, and hip. And the hip, knee, and ankle.

DIRECTIONS

- Start by placing the short edge of a yoga mat against the wall. Place your hands on the wall and your feet back. The ideal way to do this is to create an upside-down "L" shape using your legs and torso.
- Hold hands against the wall, then pull hips back
- Gently pull the navel towards the spine, encircling the center
- Arms are level with ears.
- This allows us to determine the areas where our bodies require adjustments.

WALL SQUATS

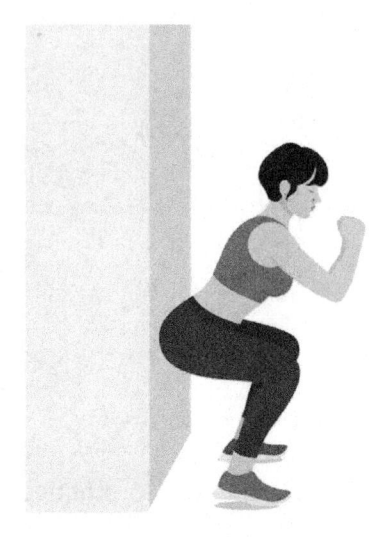

This workout targets the glutes, quadriceps, and hamstrings, and you perform it by standing with your back against the wall and feet shoulder-width apart. Use the wall as support when you squat to work your core and lower body, which will help burn fat.

For wall squats, perform 2–3 sets of 30–60 seconds. Choose a time length that allows you to maintain good technique throughout each set.

DIRECTIONS

- Stand with your back against a wall and walk. Bring both feet forward until they are shoulder-width apart, with knees over ankles. Slide back until your thighs parallel the floor; knees should overpass ankles.
- Evenly distribute your weight while gripping the floor with both feet to create a stable support base. Your upper body and head should be resting against the wall.
- Pre-tension your hips and shoulders while engaging your core. Keep your arms by your sides or place your hands on your legs. All repetitions should begin from this starting position.
- While maintaining your alignment and full-body tension, hold the wall squat position for your desired length.
- Stand up, stretch, and repeat for your desired number of sets.

WALL LUNGE

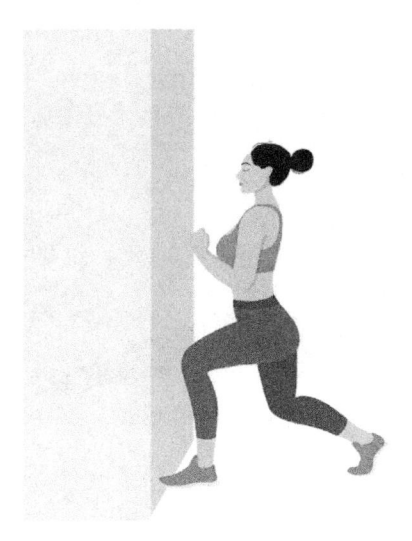

We lunge pretty frequently during our daily lives! We might not think of these movements as lunges.

Drop a pencil? It is possible to kneel to pick it up! Have you seen a friendly dog? You could take the air to greet it!

Lunges aren't easy to master. It is possible to overcome this issue by focusing on the ranges of movement we can use. This is a great way to begin!

DIRECTIONS

- It would help to have your legs approximately shoulder width apart and your hips in front.
- Ensure your heel stays on your leg on the ground to the floor. If your heel is inclined to move up, that's fine! It'll become easier over time.
- You can move your arms in any way you want to be able to balance the exercise. It's not that important.
- Do not simply run through these. Find a rhythmic, controlled speed to feel the movement. 2 Seconds Down, 1 Second Pause, 2 Seconds Up. Repeat.
- Make sure that your back stays straight throughout the exercise. This means that you should not turn or incline your back. It may take some effort in case you're not accustomed to this. However, you'll be able to progress with time.

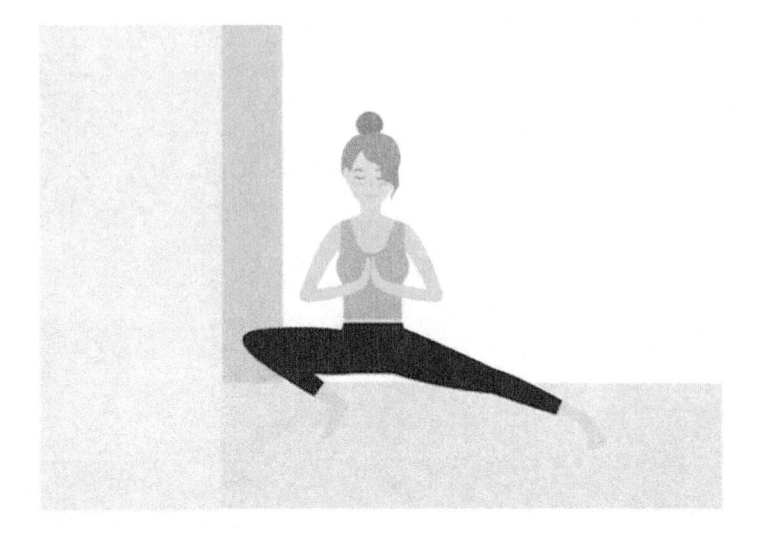

WALL SIDE LUNGE

Side lunges, also known as lateral lunges, are among my absolute favorite exercises for the legs that are bodyweight. While they might appear fairly easy at first glance, they're challenging for many people because they require lots of leg strength, flexibility, and balance to perform them correctly.

Before my passion for fitness took shape, I would have given you an ineffective and awkward exercise when you wanted me to perform the side lunge. My strength and flexibility were absent when I did the slightest lunge! However, these exercises provide an array of amazing benefits, so it's worth the effort to develop these exercises:

These exercises will help build leg strength without the need for equipment. They're an excellent opportunity to prepare for pistols since they work on balance and flexibility and make you work different motions - ideal for mobility and joint health!

DIRECTIONS

- Make two large steps to either side. As your legs become larger, the higher you'll have to take a step. Begin gently and slowly lower as you keep your legs straight. Note how your toes point slightly towards the outside on legs that are not working!
- Step back from a chair as long as you can on one leg while maintaining your other leg straight. Ultimately, the objective should be to connect your back leg with your calf muscles.
- Reverse to the beginning position by driving using your foot on the working leg. Make sure you push through your heel and the ball of your foot when you do this. Make sure that your knee isn't wobbling while doing this exercise.
- You can alternate all reps on the same leg before switching to doing them on the next leg.

WALL BRIDGE

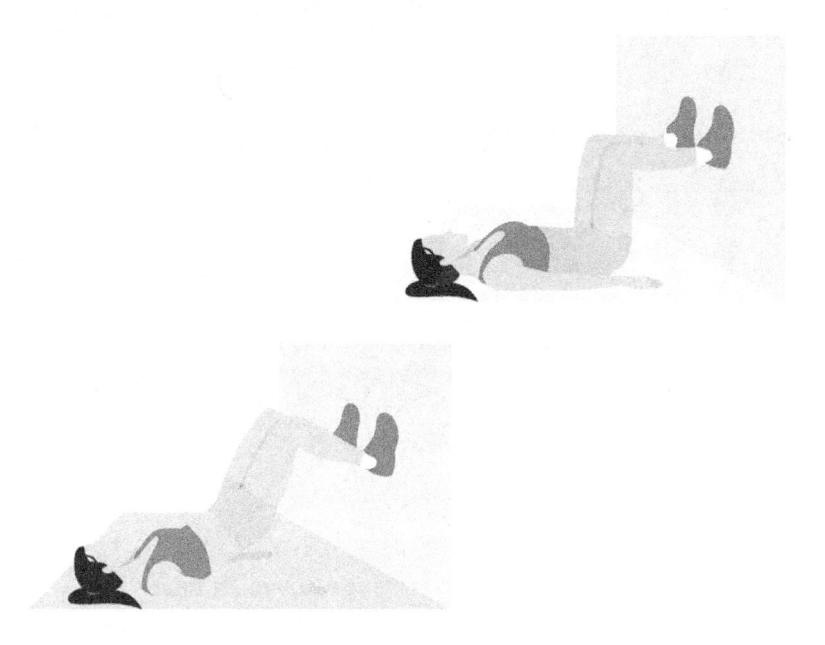

The Wall Bridge is an advanced version of the glute bridge exercise designed to target and strengthen glutes specifically. Additionally, this exercise improves the hip range of motion, increases circulation, tones your core and thighs, and improves the hip range.

DIRECTIONS

- Begin lying on your back with arms at your sides.
- Place the soles of both feet against a wall with hip-width apart feet hip-width apart, knees bent at 90-degree angles, legs at 90-degree angles and perpendicular to the floor, with your thighs perpendicular to the floor.
- Squeeze your glutes tightly as you raise your hips as far as possible.
- Return to the starting position and continue until all sets have been completed.

Proper Form and Breathing Pattern

To maintain proper form and breathing pattern, engage your core while breathing out through your nose as you squeeze your glutes to lift your butt off the floor, keeping the upper body relaxed as you return to starting position.

Sets And Reps

Once on the floor, using a wall can take this exercise to another level. To effectively engage your glutes, hamstrings, and core muscles, lie on your back with your hips against the wall in a bridge position while lifting your legs towards your chest in alternate steps.

WALL QUAD STRETCH

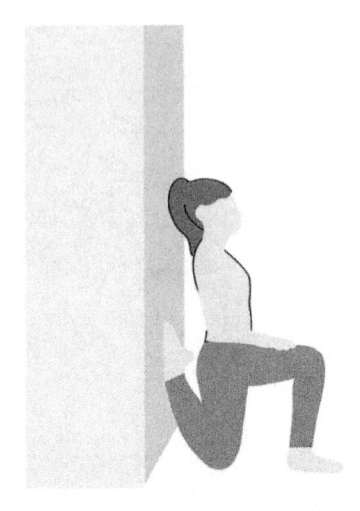

This stretch always brings to mind someone warming up for an early morning run, so I know it must be effective and straightforward in its execution. In particular, its simplicity makes it perfect for warming up before hitting the trails!

DIRECTIONS

- Start standing on one leg, using your side against a wall for balance if necessary, and placing one hand on it for extra help.
- If needed for additional balance support, bend your outside leg backward while reaching behind to grab its foot and pull toward you until a good stretch has been felt in front of the thigh.
- Hold for 30-60 seconds on either side before repeating. In between sides, stand straight and tall with abs pulled tight against your body.
- Keep your knees close together.

PUPPY STRETCH

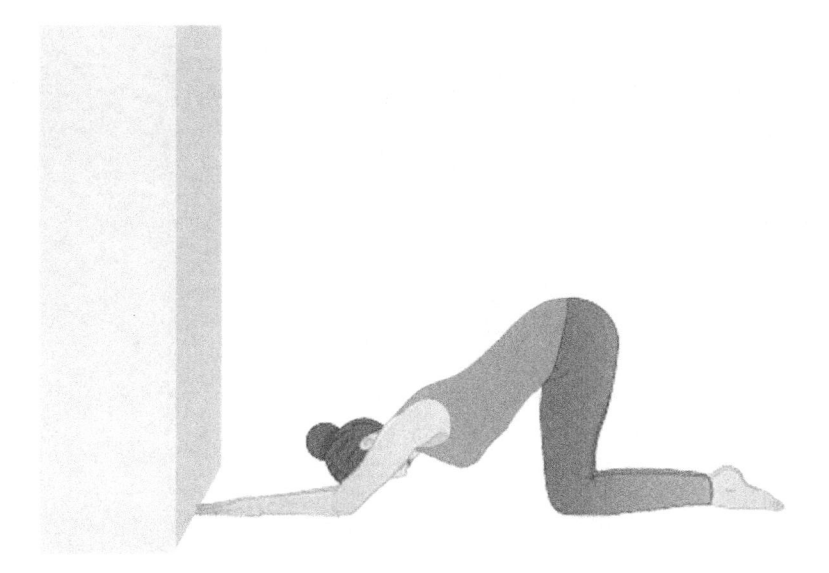

Puppy Stretch is a deep backbend designed to open your chest (and heart chakra) and stretch all areas that affect posture. When your back arches more, the front opening will increase, allowing the center chakra of your heart to open further and improve posture!

This posture is a great shoulder stretch. In addition, the abdominals and arms will experience gentle stretching while you let go of all the tension in your shoulders and back.

The puppy is inverted. That means you need to keep your heart at a higher level above your head than its top. Inversions offer many advantages to your health, like improved blood circulation, stress reduction, and general Zen.

They're a relaxing and simple way to restore harmony to your mind and body!

DIRECTIONS

- Begin in a child's position or tabletop posture and bring your knees in a straight line by placing your hands resting on the floor.
- Step forward and slide your hands to your chest on the mat. Then, lift your hips towards the ceiling, stretch your chest, and bend inwards.
- Keep in the pose briefly before moving to a different posture.

Tips and modifications:

Make sure you warm up before your workout by performing cat-cow backbends. Breathing deeply will allow you to bend further!

Modify: Place a piece of block on your forehead in case you require additional assistance to climb onto the mat. Alternately, try placing a bolster or blanket under your knees to support the knees if they are uncomfortable.

SUPINE WALL TOE TAPS

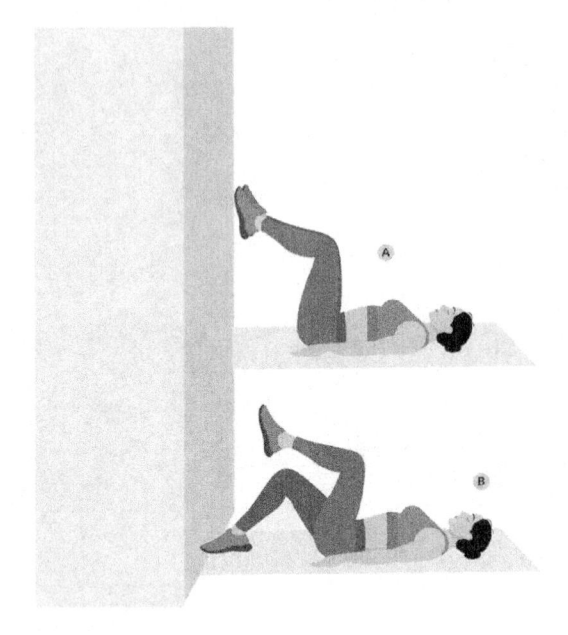

This Supine Alternate Toe Tap Exercise is designed to build and strengthen your lower back's abdominal muscles to help support your lower back.

DIRECTIONS

- To begin, lay on a mat with bent knees on the floor.
- Put your fingers on your abdominal muscles in the lower part of your back near your hip bone so you can feel them when they contract.
- Now, lift both knees toward the ceiling in preparation for this activity.
- Gently lower one foot toward the floor and touch its toes against it before slowly raising it again.
- Repeat steps 2-5 until both feet touch the floor at least twice each.
- Alternate sides as necessary. When necessary.

TIPS

- Ensure you don't let your back arch slip off its support surface when you raise your knee. Avoid putting the weight of your foot when you put it down on the floor. Finally, try to avoid holding your breath.

STANDING SIDE LEG RAISE

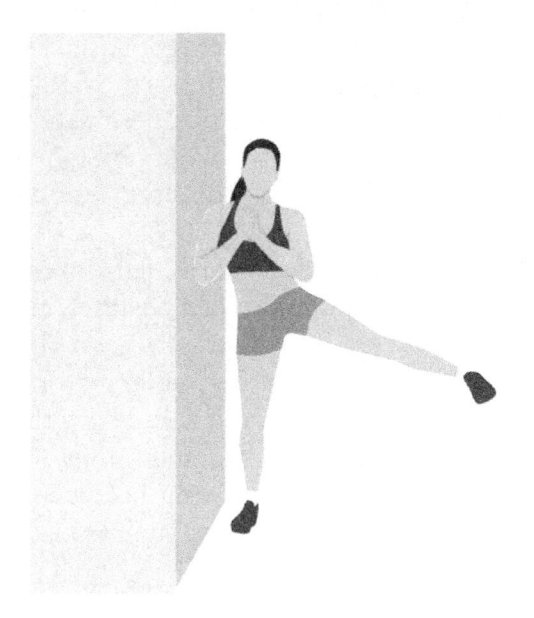

The name of the exercise sums it up. A side leg raise that you stand on is a type of exercise that requires you to raise one leg toward the opposite side. It can help strengthen your hips, buttocks, and thigh muscles. It's great for gaining better balance.

The leg that is raised from the side while standing exercise is designed to target these muscles:

Glutes. The three muscle groupsthe gluteus maximus, gluteus medius, and gluteus minimus -are all located inside your butt. The most significant one is called your gluteus maximus. However, all three muscles work to extend, rotate, and adduct your leg. They also help to pull it towards the side and assist in stabilizing your pelvis.

Quadriceps. This muscle group runs along the side of your thighs. It comprises four muscles: the vastus medialis vastus lateralis, the vastus intermedius, and the rectus fascia. It's a large muscle group -- larger than any other group of muscles within your body. Your quads play a significant role in running, walking, jumping, climbing stairs or moving to and from the seat, and squatting to pick things up off the ground.

The hip flexors. The hip flexors are on top of your pelvis between the hip bones. They comprise the iliopsoas and the rectusfemoris muscles. They aid in flexing your hip joint whenever you put on shoes and socks or walk up stairs, sit or stand, and walk over objects on the ground.

The leg raises you to do while standing exercise is a great way to enhance your daily performance in various ways. It helps strengthen and stabilize the muscles of your lower limbs. Here's a brief overview of the benefits:

Improved stability. Any exercise you do with a single leg, even if you're grabbing onto something for stability, can help enhance joint health, strength around joints, and proprioception, the body's ability to perceive its location in space. These elements improve your balance and reduce the chances of falling and injury.

- **Lower risk of falling.** Standing side leg raises can increase strength, mobility, and balance, an array of advantages that reduce the risk of falling. A study, for instance, released in Plos One, found that abductor strength (which permits you to walk sideways and raise your leg towards the other side) decreased by 1.3 percent per year between late adulthood and early. However, you can reverse these natural declines. Activities such as the side leg raise will increase strength and flexibility. The muscles with which it is performed are crucial for fall prevention. Therefore, exercising them regularly can keep you standing up.
- Increased ability to locate comfortable postures. This exercise is a solution to sitting in uncomfortable postures for too long and other postures in your life that could result in pain and aches.
- Reduced lower back pain. Balance on one leg while performing this exercise will require you to engage the core muscles. A strong core is linked with lower back pain.
- Easier daily movement. Being more flexible and strong allows you to walk on uneven terrain or step to the side to avoid falling off your balance more easily. It's also beneficial for sports that require you to move side-to-side, such as basketball, soccer, or tennis.

DIRECTIONS

- It would help if you stood with one of your sides facing a solid surface, such as a table or countertop, and then placed your hands on it to help you balance.
- The other leg should be lifted towards the side (not straight up towards the ceiling).
- Concentrate on tightening your glute and hip muscles while you stop at the top of the movement.
- Lower your leg until it is back to its starting position.
- When you complete each repetition, you'll feel your hip, thigh, and butt muscles exercising.
- Every person is different, and you might need to alter this exercise to suit your needs.

WALL SITS WITH ONE LEG EXTENDED

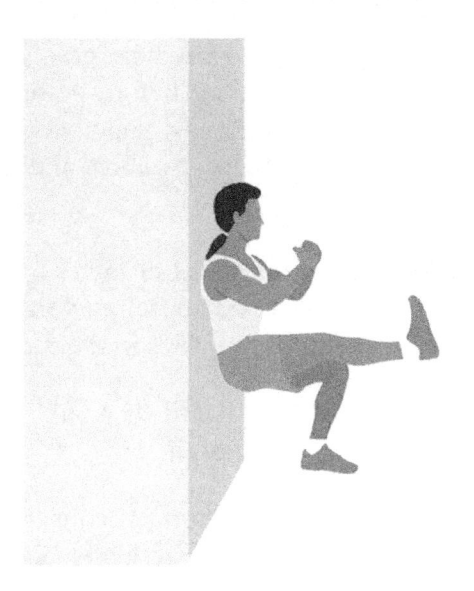

Wall sits, or wall squats, are an isometric exercise designed to target the quads, glutes, calves, and core. Although seemingly straightforward in theory, wall sits are an intensely challenging workout! Although it looks straightforward in theory, wall sits are anything but easy in practice!

Isometric exercises involve contracting muscles to build strength, endurance, and stability while managing blood pressure. Since isometric exercises don't involve moving joints directly, wall sits are excellent for arthritis patients or those recovering from an injury.

Are You Searching For an Alternative to Squatting (The Wall Sit) or Want a Unique Lower Body Exercise to Add To Your Workout Plan (Low Back Sits)? The wall sit is an effective and versatile lower body exercise for anyone wanting to develop size stability and strength in the lower body.

Wall Sits can be held or continuously performed, engaging the lower body and abdominals with each repetition.

DIRECTIONS

- For this exercise, stand with your back against a wall and position both feet at a hip-width distance apart.
- Assuming your hips are lower, adjust them until your thighs are parallel with the floor and knees are stacked above ankles, keeping your core engaged while your back, glutes, and head are flat against the wall.
- Upon reaching this position, extend the right leg so it is parallel with the floor before holding this position for the desired duration.
- Return your foot to the floor and repeat on the other side.

SUPINE WINDSHIELD WIPERS

The windshield wiper pose is a favorite amongst many who practice Yoga. Aside from its many benefits, it is a pose that feels good! Every morning before getting out of bed, this pose is an effective way to stretch and rejuvenate. By stretching your back after a lazy night's rest and gradually awakening your senses, this pose helps awaken and energize you gradually and supports a quick awakening process.

The windshield wiper pose is an effective stretch for your lower back. Slowly rotating your legs to either side of your body creates a gentle twist and stretch in your lower back muscles, creating more flexibility in your spine that may help avoid injuries in the future.

A lot of people are rigid when they only move forward. It would help to exercise your spine in various directions in a controlled environment to stay fit.

The windshield wiper posture can also help strengthen your core's oblique and transverse abdominus muscles. Turning your side, you work your lower abs while engaging the oblique muscles to the opposite side of your back. While the side turns, it is lowered, and the weights on your legs are lifted. This exercise draws in the transverse abdominous (lower abs) muscles, which draw them towards your body while engaging oblique or side obliques around the edges.

DIRECTIONS

To learn the windshield wiper pose practice, follow these steps:

- Begin by lying back on your stomach while bent with both legs, your feet flat on the floor, your arms stretched towards the sides, and your hands firmly behind your head.
- Slowly lower your knees until they are on their left-hand sides and parallel to the ground on this side - look to the right side while breathing deeply before bringing your abdominals to return your knees to their original position gradually.
- Slowly lower both knees towards that side, then lay on the floor, looking left and inhaling deeply.
- Repeat the process depending on what is desired or required.

HIP OPENER

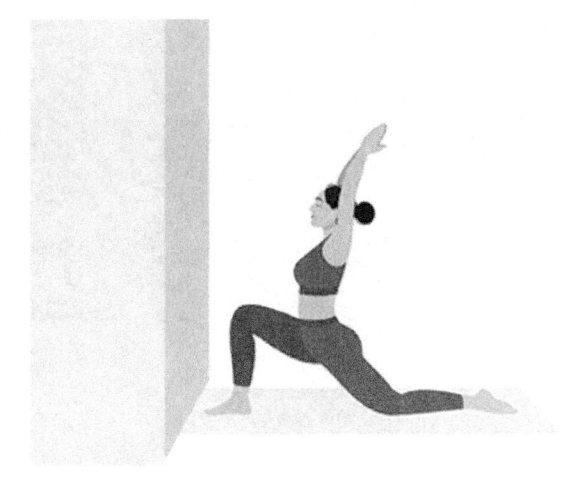

Hips don't lie; that is one great quality of theirs, but that isn't all they offer! Your hips help you walk, run, and dance! However, overusing or underusing them may cause tightness or weakness, leading to pain and physical limitations; hip openers are fantastic ways to prevent these problems and provide solutions.

DIRECTIONS

- An elastic strap will help deepen this stretch, but this opener is manageable without it as long as you remember not to lock or hyperextend your knee.
- Lie on your back with both legs extended and feet flexed.
- Slip the strap around the arch of your right foot.
- Grasp the strap in both hands, raising and pulling up on your right leg until it reaches your chest (both bum cheeks should remain on the mat while your left leg remains engaged). Hold for five slow breaths.
- Take both strap ends in your right hand, and move your right leg sideways and then down to the floor to your right (keep your hips secured to the mat. The left arm may be placed in a T or Cactus position if you wish.) Take five deep breaths.
- Return your right leg towards the center of your body and then change the strap to your left hand.
- Pull across your body toward your left side toward the floor towards your left (your arm can form T or C cactus positions if desired) until reaching the floor on your left side; hold for five slow breaths (five breaths total for this trio of exercises). When done on both legs, repeat.

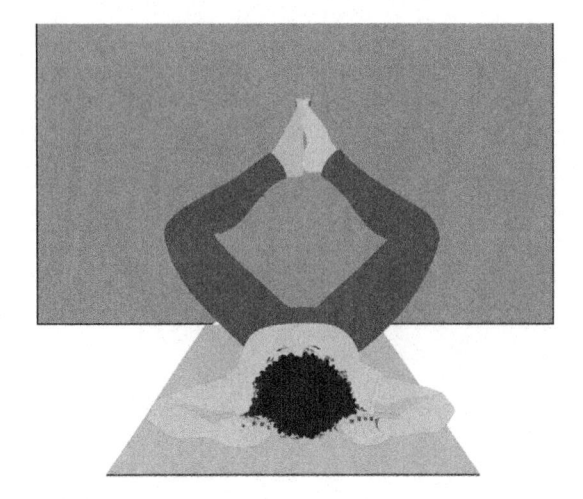

WALL BUTTERFLY

Butterfly Pose can increase flexibility and reduce tension, making it an excellent way to stretch tight hips caused by prolonged sitting or intense workouts. Furthermore, this pose promotes calmness while increasing inner awareness.

Butterfly Pose is suitable for all levels and useful in most yoga routines, making it a great starting or ending pose.

Place your feet at the edges of the cushion or folded blanket. This will give you more comfort and make standing upright while in this posture easier.

Make sure your feet are closer to your hips to intensify stretching. To maximize comfort, place cushions or blocks beneath the knees or thighs. Place your body against the wall to provide support for your spine.

DIRECTIONS

- Start in a seated place. Slowly bend your knees and press the soles of both feet to each other.
- Connect your fingers to either the pinkie-toe or heel side of your feet or put your hands on your ankles or shins to assist.
- The length and width of the chest. Pull shoulders back in place and lengthen the spine.
- Keep this position for a maximum of 5 minutes.
- To let this pose go, bend both legs in front and return your hands to your hands to release the pose.

GLUTE BRIDGE WITH KNEE TUCKS

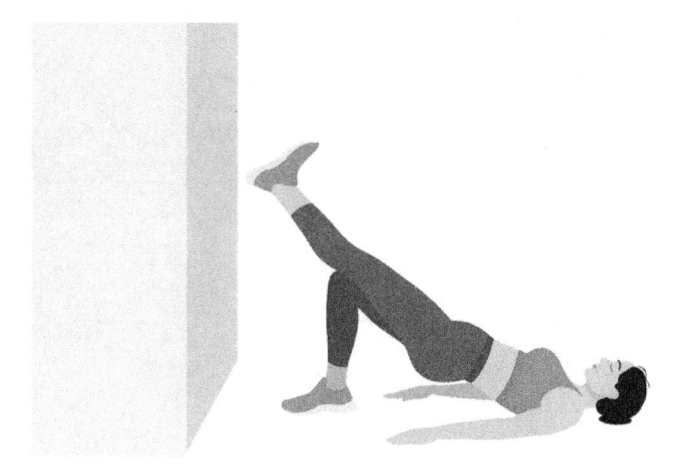

The glutes can become underactive after hours of sitting at your desk, behind the wheel, and on the couch. Over time, our bodies adapt to sitting for long hours, leading to back pain, tightness, and ineffective movement patterns.

One way to combat this issue (in addition to breaking up sitting time) is incorporating glute bridging into your workout regimen. Glute bridging exercises have long been used as an effective way of activating glutes and building core stability; plus, they require no equipment.

DIRECTIONS:

- Lie on your back with bent knees and feet flat on the floor.
- Position your feet so they are hip-width apart with toes pointed forward; the heel should be 6-8 inches away from the gluteus area.
- Place arms by your sides with palms towards the ceiling.
- Squeeze your abs and glutes as you lift your hips toward the ceiling. Raise them as high as possible without arching your back; your goal should be for your body to be straight from knee to hip and shoulder.
- Squeeze your glutes as tightly as you can while holding for two seconds in the top position while maintaining tension in your glutes and abs as you lower the hips to the floor.
- Lower your legs slowly to their original position while retaining tension in your glutes and abs.

Like most exercise routines, this focuses more on your glutes than any other muscle group. If your hamstrings are the hardest muscles, bring your feet closer to your glutes for better outcomes.

If your lower back muscles appear to be working, return to your starting posture and adjust yourself so you have your hips folded beneath. You have your abdominals in a good position when lifting your hips; ensure you maintain your core in a neutral position to avoid arching your lower back.

GLUTE BRIDGE WALKS

Finding exercises that work multiple muscles for a balanced body is important. One awesome exercise that does just that is the Glute Bridge Walk. It helps make your hip, hamstrings, and core stronger. It also improves your posture and decreases the likelihood of being injured.

Glute Bridge Walk is an easy workout suitable for all, regardless of your fitness level.

DIRECTIONS

- For the first time, start lying on your back and down with your knees bent and your feet placed flat on the floor.
- Knees should be bent slightly to lower feet until they are in the most comfortable position of sitting on the floor with palms towards the ground. Use your heels to drive your hips toward the ceiling.
- Work your core muscles.
- Slowly move your feet towards your body as long as you can.
- Take a moment to rest in this position for a few seconds.
- Move your feet back to your hips.
- Repeat the entire procedure.

BENEFITS ABOVE THE GLUTES

The addition of the Glute Bridge Walk into your workout routine will provide a variety of advantages:

Stronger Muscles: This helps to make your hamstrings, hips, and core more powerful. This will help you get more fit and perform better in sports.

Improved Posture, Less Injury The exercise will strengthen your lower body and the core muscles. Your body stays in good shape, reducing the risk of back injuries and pain.

Toning and Weight Loss Workouts on your lower and hip muscles can help you lose weight and tone up. It also helps to get rid of more calories.

The Specific Muscle Focus workout concentrates on specific muscles. This means that you can improve at other exercises and daily routine activities.

Safety First Tips and Precautions

Form and Technique: Press your hips at the top while keeping your stomach tight. This will make the exercise efficient.

Common Mistakes: Remember to work your core! Maintain your posture to get the most out of your workout.

Modifications: If you're struggling with injuries or can't make the standard move, you can do only one leg or put a bandage on to support your leg.

MARCHING GLUTE BRIDGES

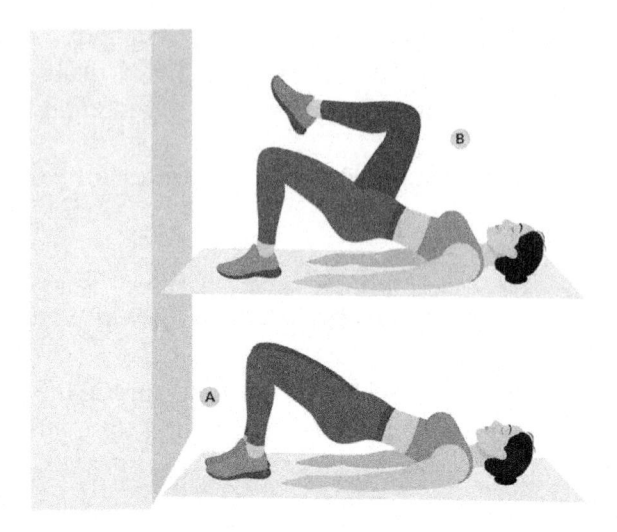

Here's another move that fires up your legs and works deep into your glute muscles. The first step is to use a wall bridge; that is an exercise.

DIRECTIONS

- Lay on your back and place your tush approximately ten inches away from the wall. Your hips and knees must be bent slightly over 90 degrees.
- Put your bottom feet into the wall, then move your hips upwards into the glute bridge. You'll see that your flexibility isn't as wide as when you utilize the floor for resistance; it's normal.
- Move one foot from the wall to the other when holding the contraction. It should appear as being along the wall.
- Do several repetitions, keeping the isometric contract in your hips, before taking a break and attempting to do it again.

ALTERNATE DONKEY KICKBACKS

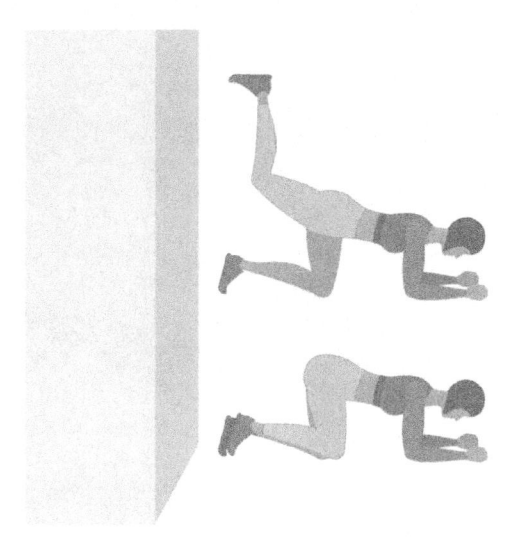

Beginning students should opt for the classic version of this exercise. Concentrate on form to ensure your back doesn't sag while your glute does all the work.

DIRECTIONS

- To begin this exercise on all fours: knees hip-width apart and hands under shoulders while maintaining neutral neck and spine alignment.
- Start by bracing your core, and lift your right leg by keeping its knee bent, foot flat, and hip hinging forward.
- Utilize the glute to press your foot directly toward the ceiling while simultaneously squeezing at its highest point; maintain pelvic alignment by ensuring the working hip stays pointed towards the ground until all movements have been completed successfully, then return to the initial starting position.
- Complete 20 repetitions on each leg for five or six sets

REACH THROUGH CRUNCH

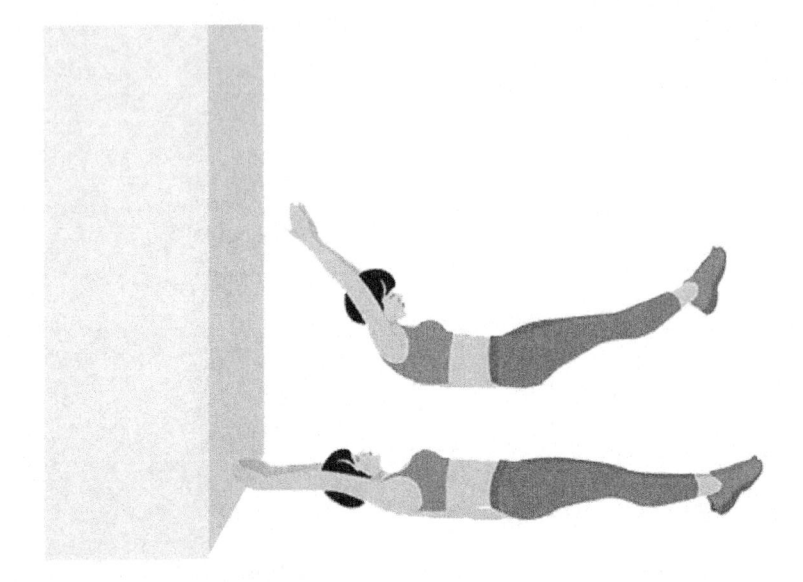

The reach crunch is a bodyweight core exercise that involves keeping the arms raised toward the ceiling while performing a crunch.

DIRECTIONS

- Spread a mat or towel out on a flat surface. Bend your knees until they reach 90 degrees, drawing in your legs by bending them in.
- Leave enough space between your legs so your arms can easily reach in and reach between them.
- Over your shoulders, reach up by lifting your arms.
- Start by seated in this posture, bringing your belly button towards the floor to activate your abdominal muscles (abs) to do the sit-up.
- Reach your arms between your legs and feet while taking breaths to create an upright position. Then, lower to the floor and repeat.
- Maintain your feet on the ground throughout your movements to avoid the temptation to place them on top of something or request anyone else to hold them so that you can utilize the legs.

CHAPTER 4
ADVANCE EXERCISE

For people who are more advanced with solid skills, using the wall, like when doing wall sits, can make them more intense. The wall might be a tool that will make your workout simple or make it more challenging, based on your preference.

WALL PLANK

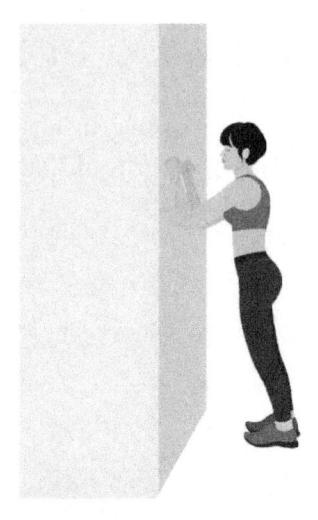

A wall plank is an alternative kind of exercise that works out your entire body. It focuses extensively on your abs, chest, calves, forearms, shoulders, hip flexors, obliques, and triceps all at once.

No matter your level, plank exercises offer multiple ways to add this challenging workout to your practice. If you want a less daunting start point and want to strengthen and lose belly fat faster, start by holding wall planks before gradually increasing their hold time.

DIRECTIONS:

- Begin by putting your hands and knees in front of a wall while you straight your arms
- Now, put the soles of your feet on the wall, ensuring your body is horizontal to the ground.
- Now, tighten your core and keep the body in a straight line
- Try keeping in this position for as long as you want.

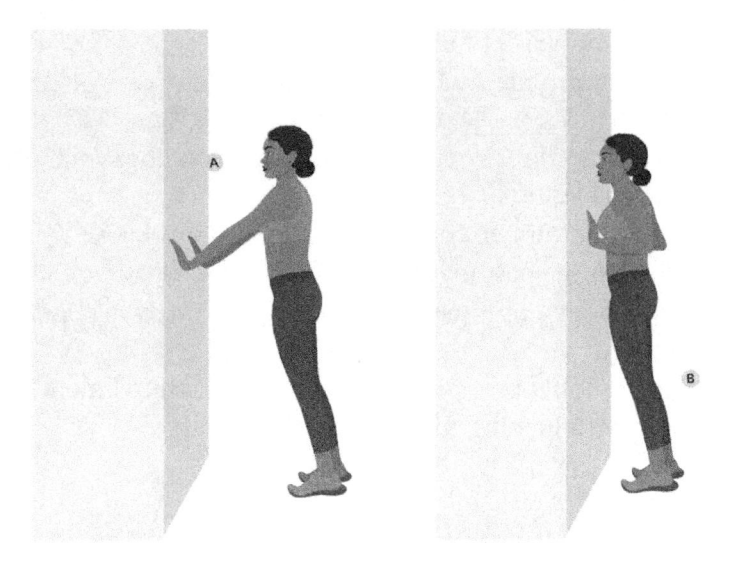

WALL PUSHUP

Wall pushups are a kind of workout that utilizes your body weight to work your chest, arms, shoulders, and muscles. Stand in front of the wall with your feet and shoulder width apart and your hands touching the wall.

Lean a little bit forward, keeping your legs and back straight, and bend your elbow to start the wall pushup.

For toning and strengthening your muscles, arms, shoulders, and chest, do some wall push-ups. Stand at a distance facing the wall, press yourself against the wall, and engage your shoulder, chest, and triceps. Remember, you need to tighten your core for stability.

Doing wall pushups frequently has numerous advantages:

- Wall pushups are easier than standard pushups. Your standing posture during wall pushups puts less strain on your shoulder joints and arms than traditional pushup posture, which involves planking on the ground.
- Wall pushups build upper-body strength. Like classic pushups, wall pushups engage muscles across your upper body, including the pectoral muscles, anterior deltoids, and triceps.
- Wall pushups increase stability. With proper form, wall pushups activate the stabilizer muscles in your midsection, including your abdominal and lower back muscles.

DIRECTIONS

Perform 2–3 sets of 15–20 repetitions for wall pushups. Choose your number of sets and repetitions following your ability to maintain proper technique.

- Begin by standing at arm's length from the wall.
- Place both hands on the wall at the same elevation as your shoulder, just a bit broader than your shoulders.

- Take a step backward with both feet. Your legs should be straight. Ensure you keep your weight on the balls of your feet.
- Rotate your shoulders outward to involve your lats.
- Squeeze your quads and glutes while engaging your core. All repetitions should begin from this position.
- Lower your chest in the direction of the wall by bending your elbows. Your shoulder blades should retract as you move.
- Lower your body till your upper arms are parallel to your back
- Pause for one second at the bottom of the activity.
- While maintaining your alignment, move upward by squeezing your chest and straightening your elbows.
- Your shoulder blades should protract as you push to the movement's top.
- End each repetition by tightening the chest and triceps.

WALL PIKE

If you think normal push-upsare a little bit challenging, don't worry! Pushups are basic exercises that will build your strength and improve your general fitness. Physical therapist value them because of their versatility and because they can be done anywhere. Moreover, there are many versions you can try, like trying out a pike pushup or doing them on your knees.

The pike pushup is an alternative to the normal pushup, providing different benefits for numerous joints and muscles. This exercise focuses on the deltoids, triceps, and core muscles. It increases blood flow to these areas, which can help in easing muscle soreness and help with fast recovery. Constant engagement of these muscles can also improve flexibility, muscle tone, and balance and reduce strain on closed joints.

Basically, a pike pushup is like a revised pushup that provides additional care to your shoulders. It works the muscles in your shoulder, most especially the front and side parts. This exercise is a good way to toughen the upper torso and enhance the complete muscle tone.

Benefits of Pike Pushups

Pike pushups, like several other bodyweight exercises, provide various health benefits, including:

- - helping in boosting the shoulder strength
- - helping to boost the core stability, enhance balance and coordination
- It improves the posture.
- Provide better functional strength, making sure day activities are easy.
- It boosts the metabolic process as muscles are metabolically active tissue.
- It improves bone density due to the weight resulting from doing the exercise
- It improves the joint health and mobility

the above benefits help you with most tasks like lifting objects above your head, carrying heavy loads, pushing objects, seeking for comfortably, driving a car, and reaching for things (like when you are painting or washing windows)

DIRECTIONS

- Get on your knees and hands and move into the downward position by widening your arms and legs and moving your in-between your arms.
- Then, gradually bend your arms to bring your head down near the ground between both hands.
- Now, straight your arms to go back to the first position.
- You will notice your arms, shoulders, muscles, and neck working during all repetitions.
- Every individual is different, so adjust the exercises to see what feels right for you.

WALL ABDOMINAL CURL

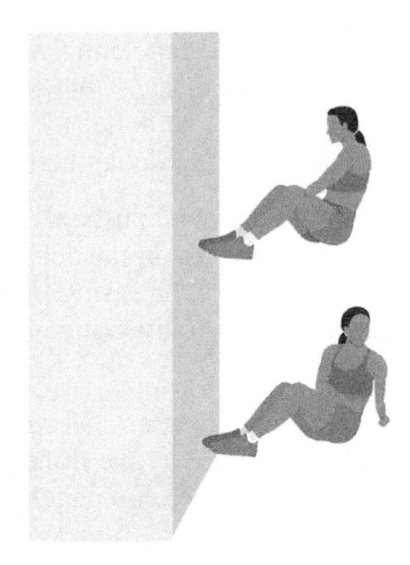

The abdominal curl is a Pilates workout that increases strength, burns calories, and tightens your core muscles, which makes it beneficial for losing weight. Doing this exercise every time will help mold your whole body and tighten the part around your stomach. You need to keep in mind that abdominal curls won't exactly burn belly fat, but they contribute to building a solid core, which enhances balance and stability.

A strong and stable body improves your stamina and endurance during workouts, making sure you burn some amount of calories during your weight loss journey.

DIRECTIONS

- Lay down on your back flat and bend your knees to complete the abdominal curl.
- If you are not able to bend your knees, place a small ball below them.
- Pull yourself upward by using your abdominal muscles to slightly curl your shoulder and upper torso off the ground.
- Avoid lengthening your neck by concentrating your eyes on the point where the ceiling and wall meet.
- Now, breathe in as you raise your body off the floor, then breathe out as you bring it back down.
- When you are done with the abdominal curl, concentrate on strengthening your belly button.
- Make sure you work on your abs instead of raising your body off the ground. If you lift yourself when your hands are at the back of your neck, you might risk hurting your neck and using little energy in your abdominal muscles. You shouldn't get back pain when you perform the abdominal curl with the right technique. If you have back pain, ensure you bend your knees and that you are pushing your belly firmly while curling your body upward with your abdominal muscles. Try avoiding arching when you are performing the abdominal curl.

If you have to sit on a balance ball to stop the back pain, then you should complete the abdominal curl in this position.

SINGLE-LEG WALL BRIDGE

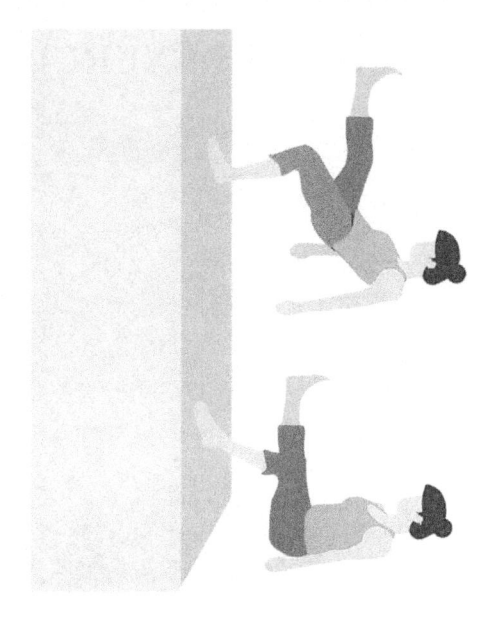

If your ground is smooth, use a fitness mat. You can put a folded towel below your shoulders if it is uncomfortable.

DIRECTIONS

- Lay on your back with one of your feet against the wall, creating a right angle, while the other leg is spread to the ceiling.
- Now, keep both arms resting next to your body.
- Then, push the foot against the wall while raising your pelvis simultaneously.
- Put your effort into keeping your arms, shoulders, and head on the floor.
- Stay in this position for about 6-10 seconds
- Now, repeat the movement by lowering your pelvis downward
- Also, don't forget to change to the other leg
- To ensure the glute exercise is comfortable, try placing the two legs against the wall.

CHAPTER 5

28-DAY WALL PILATES EXERCISE CHART

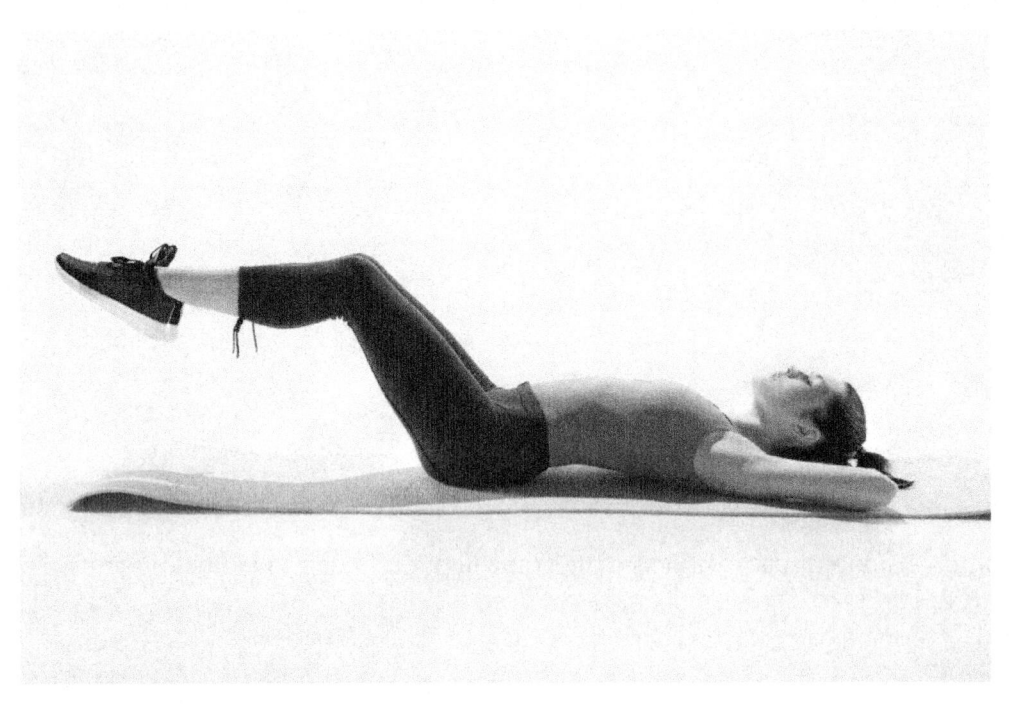

Pilates has long been heralded as a way to transform your body in appearance and strength. Until recently, however, progressing beyond basic mat work has required access to pricey studios or even pricier equipment. Luckily, wall Pilates is altering that for the better.

If you just hear about Pilates, it's a nice idea to connect in a live class with a knowledgeable trainer before trying the exercise by yourself. Proper form is necessary for getting the benefits of Pilates, just like other popular exercises.

Basic exercises are normally done using the floor, while a more advance measure include tools like the reformer, high chair, Wunda chair, and ladders barrels. Wall Pilates is another type that uses a plain wall to do different Pilates exercises, adding diversity and complexity to the routine. By adding just a wall, Pilates researchers can improve their exercises efficiently and safely without buying a lot of costly equipment and studio membership.

Wall Pilates can be beneficial in multiple ways. Although wall Pilates is related to floor Pilates, it gives extra support and firmness by utilizing walls. This provides more control and intensity to the workout. Also, it helps to develop posture and stability. Pilates is a valuable exercise option, particularly for people dealing with backaches or any postural problems, as it brings out a deeper workout with complete support.

WHAT IS (28-DAY) WALL PILATES PLAN?

This program includes some workouts from 10 to roughly 30 minutes each. The objective of the session is to work on particular areas like abs, glutes, upper body, full body, and stretching. Resting days are planned on days 7, 14, 21, and 28. Many of the routines are repetitive during the

4-week course, and some include optional equipment like dumbbells, ankle weights, a loop band, and a Pilates ball.

As we progress along the 28 days, the workout becomes more doable but can be challenging. Pilates highlights core work, helping build stability and core strength in the abdominal muscles. The 28-day Pilates program is super easy to follow, offers adjustment for people who need it and can be easily added to a busy schedule.

Twenty minutes of Pilates each day may be sufficient if performed with proper form and focus on concentrating on the primary muscles while including various movements and modifications.

Form is key when performing Pilates exercises, ensuring they target the right muscles and avoid injury occurrence. Engaging core muscles - often known as the powerhouse - also creates an efficient foundation for movement while building leaner, more toned bodies.

Integrating modifications and variations in your workout will keep your body engaged as you keep going and making great progress.

Trying out wall Pilates is an exceptional way to improve posture and alignment while strengthening important muscle groups, particularly the primary muscles. Take this guide as the first step, and stay attentive to what makes you feel at ease when you include wall Pilates into your routine.

WEEK 1: FOUNDATION BUILDING

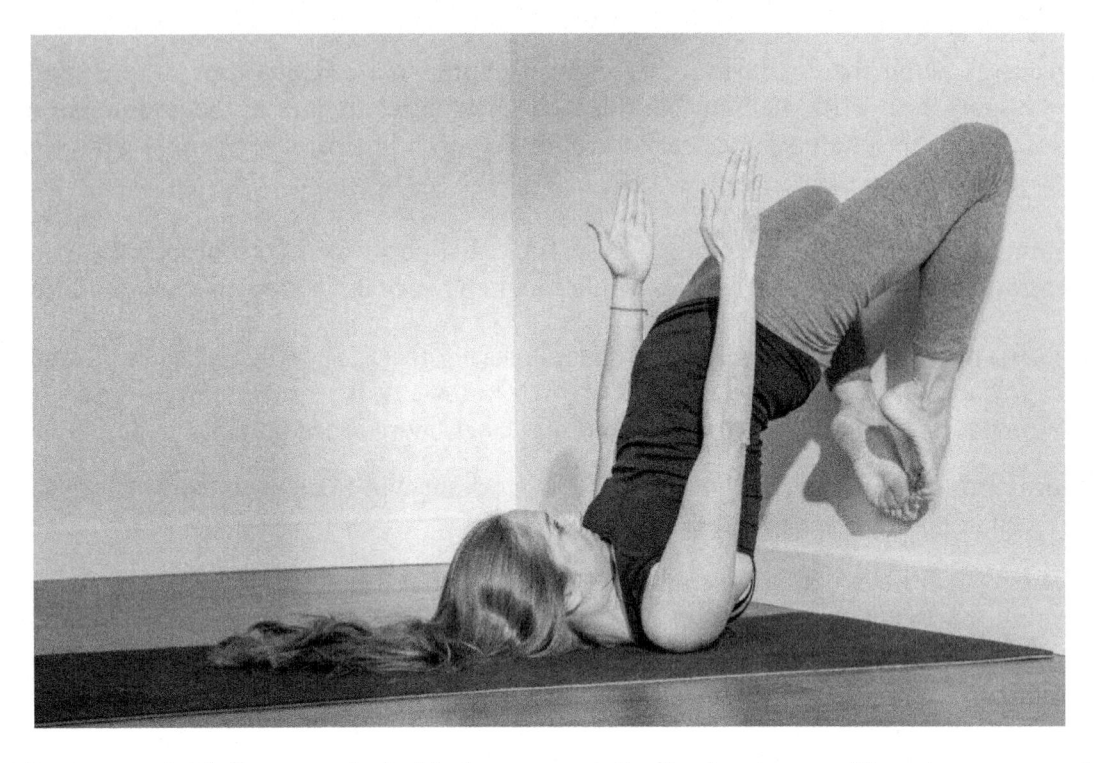

Wall Pilates may initially seem intimidating, especially for beginners. Here is an example of a full-body routine you can try:

GENTLE WALL PILATES WARM-UP

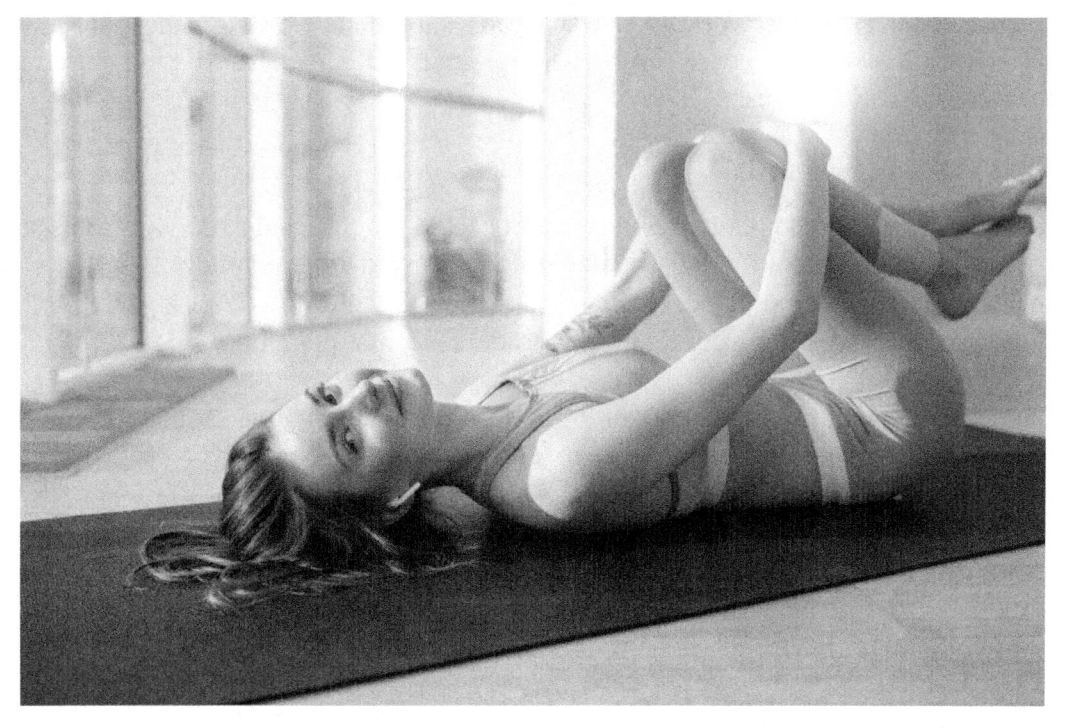

Warm-up before every Pilates session helps to avoid injury. The purpose of Pilates warm-up exercises is to prepare your body for a rigorous movement regimen. The workout in wall Pilates supports and helps in opening your joints, loosens the cartilage between both joints and ensures your muscles are flexible enough, organizing them for exertion. The warm-up is an essential part of the Pilates workout. Supposing you didn't do a complete warm-up before a session, there are many exercises you can pick from to prepare your abs for an intense workout. Here are several warm-up workouts specially designed for wall Pilates.

1. PILATES IMPRINTING

The wall Pilates imprint is an easy warm-up workout done while you lay on your back. It helps you understand your body more and steadily wakes up every muscle. Imprinting is a good way to reduce stress at any time, but it's very necessary to ensure your body is in sync before Pilates.

DIRECTIONS

- Lie down on the floor or Pilates mat, putting your back on the ground. Bend your knee and put your feet flatly on the floor, making your spine get back to its position.
- Slowly relax your shoulder, throat, mouth, belly, hips, rib cage, and leg muscles one after the other. Take a deep breath through your nose, and slowly exhale through your mouth during the complete process
- in your head; feel your spine expanding, relaxing, and stretching against the floor. The workout gets its name through the imprint your vertebrae leave on the mat.
- Keep on imprinting on your mat for 3-5 breaths.

2. ARM REACH AND PULL

Attaining success in a Pilates workout needs strong shoulders. So, it's necessary to correctly warm-up your shoulders and arms before using Pilates equipment or taking part in a deep workout during structure classes.

DIRECTIONS:

- Stand on your feet shoulder and width apart on the ground, and raise your arms straight in your front, keeping your wrist at a high point with your fingers totally free.
- Inhale and open your shoulder blade as you reach forward
- Exhale, letting your shoulders get back to their normal position while keeping your arm stretched
- Inhale once again, pulling your arms backward and making your shoulder blades meet.
- Now, exhale, letting your shoulder relax and letting your arms drop.

3. PELVIC THRUST

This simple thrusting workout, also known as the pelvic curl, lifts your pelvic a little bit from the floor, slightly involving your abdominal and leg muscles. Due to the fact that it can be demanding, you might choose to do this workout tat the end of your stretching practice.

DIRECTIONS:

- Begin with your Pilates breathing sequences
- Now, exhale and activate your abdominal muscles to lower your pelvis near the floor.
- Inhale as you lift your tailbone upward and press your feet downward. Start by raising your hips, followed by your upper and lower back.
- Now, keep it straight from your hips to your shoulder.
- Exhale, then return your pelvis to the floor, inverting the order in which you raise it.

4. WALL ROLL DOWN

The wall roll-down is a stretch that helps warm up your abdomen and activate the spine. It serves as a good changeover exercise between the floor and standing positions. Using the wall will make sure there is appropriate alignment. This exercise is easy and can be done even at home or at work for a quick boost.

DIRECTIONS:

- Stand and put your back against the wall, then walk your feet about 6-10inches away.
- Now, bend your knees if you are on a chair.
- Now, pull your bellybutton inward your spine and raise the two arms straight up over your head.
- Put your head downward, then gradually roll your spine down the wall
- Now, keep rolling up, one vertebra at a time, till you are in a straight standing position.

5. SWAN PREP

This form of the superman stretch includes raising your head without raising your feet from the ground. If you want, you can substitute it with the complete superman, where your hands are well stretched out while you raise your feet from the ground when you lift your head.

DIRECTION:

- Lay on your back, putting your hands by your sides while bending your elbow.
- Use your abs to raise your belly away from the mat as you breathe in and broaden your spine.
- Now, breathe out, gradually lowering your spine to bring back your belly to the mat.

6. SPINE STRETCH

Think about your body forming the shape of the tight letter "C." In short, that's the Pilates spine stretch

DIRECTIONS:

- Sit with your back straight while your buttocks are on the floor
- Now, spread your legs forward, a little bit wilder than shoulder-width, and put them apart
- Inhale as you raise your arms up and forward while your palms are facing down.
- Now, exhale and push your upper body forward while keeping your leg in a straight line. You should curve your spine in a "C" shape.
- Now, inhale as you lift your torso back to the starting point with an appropriate spinal movement.

Although all warm-up exercises can be helpful, the six stated above are especially important for a Pilates workout. It's best to warm up before every session, not just to avoid injury but also to get the most out of your workout.

WALL SQUATS AND LEG LIFTS

DIRECTIONS

- While your back is against a strong wall, stand up rightly. Then, slowly lower your knees so they make a right angle. Your thighs and shins should be shaped like a corner (precisely a 90-degree angle).
- Place your hands on your hips, then lift one leg up. Next, switch legs and repeat.
- Moving the leg exercises from the floor to the wall will help make your legs stronger and enhance your ability to stay balanced.
- Navigate to a plank position with your feet against the wall. Raise one leg up, then the other, to work your lower body, core, and butt muscles while keeping steady.

WALL SQUATS WITH ARM RAISES

The wall squats with arm raises incorporate the big muscles of your legs. This will help to fire up the cardiovascular portion of your wall Pilates workout. It also does a pretty good job of warming the upper part of your body up.

DIRECTIONS

- To begin this exercise, stand with your back against the wall.
- Gently move your feet forward while bending your knees till your legs make a rectangle shape under you. Ensure that your knees are bent at about a right angle (90degrees). However, if you find this difficult, you can bend them a little less. Remain in this position without moving for sometime.
- When your legs are placed in the right position, place your arms by your sides and keep your palms directly on the wall.
- Keep your arms straight, then lift them up so your fingertips touch the wall above your head. Lower them back down while remaining in the squat position.
- If you want to make things interesting, you could alter your arm movements. This will aid in taking your mind off the strength your legs are putting in. For instance, you could shift your arms out to the sides like you're trying to make a snow angel. Alternatively, you could raise them up to shoulder height, lower them into the chest, and then straighten them out again.

WALL BRIDGE EXERCISE

As you've probably experienced, glute bridges on the floor can be challenging enough. To gain a good amount of knowledge on wall glute bridges, I donned a few grippy socks to protect my paintwork. Next, I unrolled a good yoga mat and then included wall glute bridges as part of my workout for seven days straight.

If you are looking for good exercise for your backside muscles, the glute bridge is the right exercise for you. It is simple and targets your butt, hamstrings, and core. Also, if you sit a lot during the day, it could aid in stretching out your hip flexors. Here's how to do it right!

Remember, what works for me might probably not be right for you, as it may not work for you. If you're a beginner at exercising or have had an injury, it is smart to talk to a personal trainer before checking out fancier versions, like lifting your feet up on a wall.

HOW TO DO A WALL GLUTE BRIDGE

As you might have suspected, this task requires a wall. If you're not at the gym, it's generally preferable to take off your cross-teaching boots and perform this exercise in socks or barefoot. As you will likely be lying on your back, one of the top yoga mats may come in handy as an aid when resting against walls.

DIRECTIONS

- To begin with, on the back, put both arms alongside your body, pressing into the floor while walking your feet up the wall until they are hip-width apart with knees bent at 90-degree angles and perpendicular to the floor. Your thighs should also remain perpendicular.
- Squeeze your glutes, engage your core, and raise the hips towards the ceiling, pausing at the top before reverting to the beginning posture but keeping your glutes hovering until all reps have been completed.
- Leave the upper region of the body still when performing this exercise and press flat into the mat - any movement should come from your glutes alone.
- Engage your core while breathing regularly; moving slowly with control is key here - don't rush through reps!

WALL PLANKS FOR CORE STRENGTH

Wall planks can give athletes a firm foundation from which to generate power and move freely and generate movement. Achieving peak athletic performance requires having a strong core; wall planks can help strengthen this area for increased performance in various sports and activities.

Wall planks benefit your fitness routine, improving core strength, stability, and overall well-being. By including wall planks in your fitness regimen, you can reap these advantages to achieve results that transform core strength, stability, and well-being.

For an effective full-body exercise, wall planks engage the core muscles and target other groups like the deltoids, glutes, quadriceps, and erector spinae.

Wall planks can easily be tailored to accommodate different levels of fitness by altering body positioning or including different variations. Wall planks can also virtually be done anywhere there's a robust vertical section, which enables them to be accessible and convenient exercises.

1. ARM WALL PLANK

Because of this modification, the activity can now be more challenging because you can only utilize one of your arms at once. However, it will help to make sure that your balance and core work harder.

Start by assuming the standard wall plank stance. Then, take one hand off the wall very lightly and either rest it on the hip or extend it outwards toward the side.

DIRECTIONS:

- Start in the normal position for wall planks.
- Hold a one-arm wall plank for fifteen to thirty seconds, making sure to maintain appropriate form and alignment.
- Before doing the procedure again with the opposite arm, put the palm of your hand onto the wall.

2. SIDED WALL PLANK

Wall plank for the side places focus on oblique muscles for an effective core workout.

DIRECTIONS

- Try to stand upright, but face sideways to your wall. Make it approximately two to three feet away.
- Put one forearm against a wall. Make sure that the elbow is directly over your shoulder.
- Extend both legs and stack your feet leaning against the wall to create an inverted V shape with your body in front.
- Hold this position for around 30 seconds in order to engage your core. Then, swap sides and continue the workout.

3. WALL PLANK WITH LEG LIFT

For a challenging yet comprehensive workout, incorporate leg lifts into your wall plank exercise to activate your gluteal and lower back muscles.

DIRECTION:

- Start in the normal position for wall planks.
- One leg should be raised gradually off the ground whilst remaining straight and in correct alignment.
- Continue for five to ten seconds, then descend gradually.
- Unless the targeted number of repetitions is reached, repeat the procedure 2 through 8 again.

4. WALL PLANK WITH KNEE TUCKING

This variation engages lower abs and hip flexors to put your core exercise to the test.

DIRECTION:

- Start in the normal wall plank position.
- Lower one of your knees and move the knee in the direction of the chest. Do not let your hips sag or rotate, holding for approximately two to three seconds prior to reverting the foot to the floor.
- Repeat these exercises alternating between legs until reaching the chosen number of repetitions.

5. WALL PLANK WITH SHOULDER TAP

Shoulder taps add challenge to the wall plank and boost upper-body activation whilst testing your coordination.

DIRECTIONS

- Start with the wall plank stance as usual.
- Slowly raise a single hand off the wall and tap the shoulder of the person on the other side while maintaining stability and using your core.
- Prior to performing the task using the other hand, slide yourself back on the wall.
- For as many repetitions as intended, alternate hands and perform as many repetitions as desired while keeping good form and alignment during each exercise.
- It's not necessary to limit your fitness goals to distant dreams of a toned and slimmer body; incorporating wall planks into your routine has several benefits, such as:

1. **Enhanced capability of Core**

Wall planks assist you in building and maintaining your core more efficiently by working the rectus abdominis, transverse abdominis, and obliques all at once.

2. Improved Flexibility and Alignment

Wall planks force the body to stay at an angle against a wall, which improves coordination, balance, and general stabilization.

3. Enhances Posture

Wall planks assist in strengthening core muscles, which supports good spinal alignment and reduces the chance of slouching or hunching, which enhances stance.

4. Greater Adaptability

Wall planks improve the variety of motion as well as flexibility by extending and stretching a number of muscles, including the calves, hamstrings, and shoulders. They also lessen pain in the lower back.

5. Decrease in Pain in the Lower Back

Robust and balanced core muscles can relieve pressure from pain in the lower back by helping support weak core muscles and alleviate any discomfort caused by their weakness.

WALL PLANKS MISTAKES TO AVOID AND HOW TO CORRECT THEM

- Sagging Hips: This issue places stress on your lower back. To correct it, engage core muscles and ensure a straight path from head to heels.
- Picking Hips: Overexerting yourself may undermine the effectiveness of an exercise routine, so focus on maintaining a diagonal line with both core and glute activation to stay on target with this strategy.
- Dropping Head: Letting your head drop strains the neck and disrupts spinal alignment, so be mindful of maintaining a neutral head position with an inward gaze and gaze slightly downward.
- Holding Breath: Failing to breathe normally during a wall plank exercise may lead to dizziness and prevent you from holding your position effectively. Take even and controlled breaths during this exercise for maximum results.

HOW OFTEN SHOULD YOU PERFORM WALL PLANKS?

For optimal results, wall planks should be added to your workout regimen 2-3 times per week, with at least 48 hours between sessions for muscle recovery.

Wall planks should be part of a holistic fitness regimen for all muscle groups. Overdoing wall planks or any exercise may result in detrimental side effects:

Muscle Fatigue

Prolonged wall planking without taking breaks to restore muscle energy may lead to excessive fatigue, decreasing your ability to sustain proper form and increasing the risk of injury.

Overuse Injuries

Overworking muscle groups for an extended period without sufficient recovery time may result in overuse injuries such as strains, sprains, or tendonitis, resulting in decreased performance and subsequent overuse injuries. Initially, these injuries can appear minor, but over time, their impact can become severe enough that performance decreases substantially and recovery takes longer.

Reduced Activeness

Since the muscles need time to heal and gain power in order to stay more potent afterward, excess exercise can negatively impact the way you perform.

Overemphasizing a single activity or group of muscles can lead to muscular imbalances, which can worsen posture, raise the risk of injury, and impede the development of fitness.

For maximum effectiveness, while limiting overtraining risks and injuries, create an exercise routine that targets multiple muscle groups while providing enough rest and recovery time. By doing this, you can minimize risk and still get the best results.

An effective core workout that has numerous benefits is wall planking. These benefits include stronger core muscles, better posture, more flexibility, and a reduction in lower back pain.

You may attain the best benefits while lowering your risk of overtraining and injury by incorporating wall grip modifications into your physical activity at least twice per week, as well as emphasizing good form.

WALL 100S

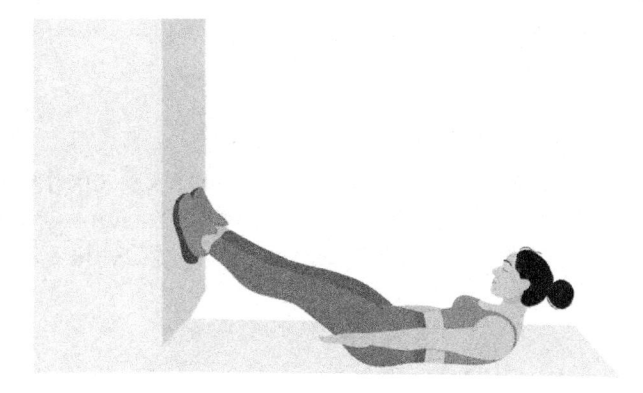

The 100s are probably the best-known Pilates core exercises. As your power increases, you can try different wall modifications.

DIRECTIONS

- To start with, lie on your back and create a rectangle beneath your knees, similar to wall squats.
- Knees and hips should bow at around 90° degrees. Rotate your head, shoulders, and upper back off the floor while contracting your abdominal muscles.
- Take fast breaths while extending your fingertips toward your feet and pushing downward.
- To add diversity to this motion, shift your feet. You can increase the angle of your knees. You may also incorporate a combination move by doing one wall glute bridge after doing a set of 100s.

WEEK 2: INTERMEDIATE WALL PILATES MOVES

SIDE LEG RAISES ON THE WALL

DIRECTIONS

- Lie comfortably on your back, face a wall, with legs stretched vertically and arms spread beside. With your heels resting against the wall, lift each leg individually at about 45-degree angles toward your body until both reach equal levels.
- Alternate for 20 repetitions.

WALL PILATES PUSHUPS

It is time to train the upper part of your body. Wall push-ups engage your triceps, biceps, chest, and shoulders.

The wall allows you to adjust the angle of the inclination with pushups, rendering it easier to use or thrilling according to your demands.

DIRECTIONS

- Start by stepping a foot or more off the wall. Put both hands exactly parallel to the center of your chest. Lean your body weight forward as if the wall were the floor, and do a typical pushup.
- You may employ diversity here as well. Do you desire to check your balance? Perform a one-armed wall pushup. Once you've mastered that motion, do a leg raise with the opposing leg. You have the sensation of your upper body working now.
- Experiment with different hand positions. Putting them broader with the elbows extended stresses your chest and shoulders, whilst drawing them in and maintaining your elbows narrow targets your triceps more.

WEEK 3: ADVANCED WALL PILATES CHALLENGE

WALL PIKE EXERCISE

The pike push-up may assist in developing amazing power and has a similar appearance to the downward-facing dog and dolphin positions.

Use it as a stepping-stone towards more challenging moves or as an exercise goal to build shoulder strength. Ensure you keep good form to protect your shoulders and avoid face-planting!

The pike push-ups constitute a formidable exercise to build shoulder strength. Every rep of this exercise will wring every bit of strength from your upper body - particularly your shoulders! Though similar to traditional push-ups, its inverted V shape emphasizes the shoulders more than the chest.

Prepping yourself for a handstand begins by perfecting the classic push-up; once proficient with that movement, adding pike push-ups as an alternate exercise to build strength for a handstand or handstand push-up will only become beneficial over time.

As soon as your weight shifts into the pike position, your core must fire up to keep from toppling forward and causing injury. This advanced push-up teaches your body how to be in tune with having its weight shift overhead.

HOW TO PERFORM THE IDEAL PIKE PUSH-UP

Beginners, anybody healing from an elbow or shoulder injury, or anyone susceptible to dizziness or low blood pressure should avoid the pike push-up exercise. When doing this move, keep your form in mind and prioritize quality over quantity.

DIRECTIONS

- Begin in a plank posture, with hands on the floor and toes pressed firmly against it.
- Keep your core strong, back flat, glutes engaged, and hamstrings extended. Your entire body should create an arch.
- To produce an inverted V shape, raise your hips up and back while maintaining your arms and legs straight.
- Gently drop the upper body to the floor by bending the elbows.
- Hold the position for a time, then gently push back up to form an inverted V with your arms straight. Be sure to keep control during the movement.

WALL PILATES ROLL-UP

The Pilates Roll Up is a staple of Pilates mat classes. If you attend them regularly, you'll have performed this exercise (and variations of it) plenty of times.

This is because the roll-up is considered a basic Pilates exercise. But don't confuse "basic" with "easy." This move is a real challenge for the abdominal muscles and is much more effective than traditional crunches. Successfully achieving this exercise also requires flexibility, strength, and the coordination of breath and movement. This is not just a beginner Pilates exercise!

For the above reasons, the roll-up can be difficult to get right. Common mistakes include letting your legs lift off the ground, gripping through the hips, or relying on momentum to get you up. But by using the tips and instructions below, you'll learn how to master the Pilates Roll Up to reap the benefits.

The roll-up exercise is just what it sounds like! You start lying on the floor and roll yourself into a sitting position. However, it doesn't just end there – it could also be called the 'roll down' since rolling back down from sitting to lying is also part of the exercise and requires eccentric strength in the abdominals and hip flexors (note: eccentric means that the muscle is lengthening under tension, rather than contracting and shortening).

The roll-up differs from other abdominal exercises in combining spinal mobility, breathing control, and strength.

Many people with strong abdominals may also create a lot of rigidity in their torso and struggle with the roll-up exercise.

Tensing the abdominals hard, bracing the abdominals, or holding your breath are all strategies that prevent the spinal mobility necessary for the roll-up exercise.

HOW TO DO THE PILATES ROLL-UP

- Starting by lying on your back on the floor with straight legs and arms extended overhead in an arc until they lie flat against the floor behind you - your head should now rest between your arms.
- If you find this position uncomfortable, reduce your range of movement and keep your arms hovering above the mat.
- Inhale to prepare. Exhale and bring your arms overhead in an arc. When the arms move past 90 degrees, twist your head, neck, and shoulder blades off the mat. This part of the exercise looks like the starting position of the Pilates Hundred.
- Inhale again here and exhale as you roll up the rest of the way. Focus on the sensation of your ribs sliding towards your pelvis as you do so.
- As you roll through the spine, imagine a ball nestled in your stomach and move around it – this should help your spine find a deep, rounded shape.
- Once you've curled up, pause with your fingers stretching towards your toes, maintaining your spine in that "C" shape. Remember: don't allow your arms to drop. Instead, keep them lifted and parallel to the floor.

- Now, inhale to extend your spine from the pelvis up through your lower spine, middle spine, neck, and head until you sit on your sit bones. These are the bones in your butt cheeks.
- Exhale and roll back to the starting position.

PEOPLE WHO SHOULD AVOID THIS EXERCISE

People with acute disc pathology, acute cervical pathology, or osteoporosis.

BENEFITS OF THE ROLL-UP

If you want to strengthen your abdominals, the Roll Up is the exercise to choose. According to researchers at Auburn University in Montgomery, Alabama, the roll-up is 30 percent more effective than simple crunches. This is because of the way it targets the rectus abdominis (the six-pack muscles) and recruits more muscle fibers.

Aside from strong abdominals, the roll-up exercise effectively increases your body's flexibility by improving hip flexor length and mobilizing your spine. This is important because an inflexible body can lead to pain, making your movement less efficient. Plus, a stiff spine leaves your back vulnerable to injury. However, practicing the Roll Up can help you avoid these problems.

On top of all that, the Roll Up promotes deep breathing and better circulation. In combination with the massaging effect of the exercise on the stomach organs, this boosts your digestive system.

PILATES ROLL-UP MODIFICATIONS AND VARIATIONS.

PILATES ROLL-UP: LEGS BENT.

Performing the Pilates roll-up with the legs bent is an easier variation. You can place the hands behind the thighs as you sink into a 'C' curve, allowing you to find this shape in a supported position. If you have tight hamstrings, aka, and can't touch your toes, you will find this position much easier than the straight-leg version.

PILATES ROLL UP: LEGS STRAIGHT

The full roll-up can be performed with the legs straight. This variation can give you more leg weight to counterbalance your upper body, but it can be hard to hold the legs here. This variation is great if you tend to get a lot of tension in the strong hip flexor muscles at the hip crease.

PILATES ROLL-UP: WITH A PARTNER!

A buddy can be a great way to work on your roll-up. A partner can help you hold your feet on the floor for more stability. A partner could also assist with your arm movements – they can take you lightly by the hands and then guide your hands up, overhead, and forwards. This will let the rest of your body follow the movement of your arms and take some of the load off your abdominals.

PILATES ROLL-UP: USING A STRAP

In this variation of the roll-up, you loop a strap or a resistance band around your feet and hold both ends with your hands. This gives you lots of support to help you up as you roll up off the mat.

PILATES ROLL-UP: ON A TRAPEZE TABLE

The large Pilates equipment can help you master the Pilates roll-up. Performing the roll-up on the trapeze table is similar to having a partner assist you (and doesn't require pulling on your poor pal). Holding on to the dowel, attached to springs, gives you a helping hand to get up off the table.

PILATES ROLL-UP: ON A REFORMER

The Pilates reformer is another great way to work on your roll-up. The weight of your upper body can be supported by holding onto the reformer straps. Sitting on the moving carriage is a great way to work on the mobility of your lower back. As the carriage moves forward, it does the work of rolling you into a 'C' shape rather than you having to do the work yourself.

HOLDS AND PULSES

If you're good at the roll-up and want to add some spice, try stopping at intervals on the way down and holding for 5 seconds. If you are still not feeling the challenge – add some pulses to feel the burn.

ADD WEIGHTS

Holding dumbells in your hands as you perform the roll-up will increase the challenge and your strength.

TIPS

- The roll-up requires your pelvis to move between neutral and tilted. Despite this, you shouldn't be over-tucking the pelvis or pressing your lower back into the mat during this exercise. Doing so will make it harder to get up in the initial phase.
- Practicing pelvic tilts can improve this aspect of the exercise.
- Create a smooth curling movement of the spine by imagining a wheel turning on the side of your pelvis.
- Full inhales and exhales as you move will also make the roll-up easier.
- Lifting your legs or gripping your hips

If you find that you are over-using your hip flexors or that your legs are lifting off the ground as you move, try these three modifications.

- Take the two ends of a resistance band into your hands and loop them around the soles of your feet. Use it for support as you roll up and down.

- Bend your knees instead of making them straight during the exercise. This can stop the over-activity of the hip flexors. It is also more comfortable for those with hamstring limitations.
- With your knees bent, reach your hands to the back of the thighs. Now, use the strength of your arms to aid you as you roll up.

HOW TO MAKE THE ROLL-UP MORE CHALLENGING

Using the magic circle prop during the roll-up adds challenge and incorporates more muscles into this exercise.

Try it: add it to your Roll Up by taking the magic circle between the palms of your hands. Keep your arms straight as you gently squeeze the circle, and maintain this pressure as you roll up and down. This will engage various upper body parts, including your lats, shoulders, chest, and arms.

COMBINING MOVES FOR FULL-BODY ENGAGEMENT

Full-body workouts can help you build strength and improve your cardio and endurance. Full-body workouts are a great way to increase the intensity of your fitness routine. Strength training exercises provide benefits ranging from strength and endurance training to core stability development and cardio. Squats with overhead presses or weighted lunges are great full-body workouts you can do anywhere!

Full-body workouts differ from standard cardio or strength training routines because they encompass the entirety of one's body and provide all-inclusive results. They aid strength training, endurance, and core stability training, creating an "afterburn effect" and helping burn more calories and fat than ever!

Most full-body exercises combine several separate exercises or add weights and extra movements for a dynamic workout, necessitating more coordination than traditional weight lifting.

Mastering a full-body workout and avoiding injury requires starting slowly with low weight to perfect form and technique, gradually increasing weight and frequency as time progresses. With that in mind, here are the best full-body exercises to consider doing:

SUPPORTED ROLL DOWN (1 MINUTE).

- Stand tall against a wall. Walk your feet 6 inches away while keeping your back in contact with it.
- Brace your core by keeping your shoulders down and away from your ears.
- As you carefully roll down spine vertebra by vertebra, feel your back muscles gradually lengthen as you descend.
- Exhale when reaching the bottom of the roll while keeping arms parallel to sides.
- Hold one to two breaths before inhaling as you ascend toward your starting position.
- Repeat five more times.

HIP OPENER IN STANDING (0:45 SECONDS)

- Step up next to a wall and lean a single hand against it for stability.
- Maintaining your pelvis square and level, raise your outer leg until its thigh is parallel to the floor.
- As aid, rest your inner hand against an elevated thigh.
- When you exhale, push your lifted leg in the palm of the palm of the hand so it opens outwardly towards one side. Maintain the position for a moment or two and then inhale to bring it back to its beginning position.
- Continue on the opposite side.

SIDE LEG SWING (30 SECONDS PER SIDE).

- Start standing next to the wall with one hand on it for support, then raise one leg until its thigh is in line with the floor while keeping your pelvis level and square to the front.
- Then, swing your leg sideways as far as possible while maintaining your pelvic stability and level.
- Switch sides by swinging your leg back towards its original starting position.
- Repeat on the other side.

ACTIVE CALF STRETCHING (0:45 PER SIDE).

- Start standing next to a shoulder-high wall with your palms flat against it - hands flat against the wall.
- Step back about two feet with your left leg while keeping its heel flat on the floor.
- Bending your right knee slightly, lean into the wall until a stretch is felt in your left calf, and hold for one or two breaths before repeating and releasing on the opposite side.

SUPPORTED SEMI LUNGE

- To begin, stand next to a wall with one hand on it for support and step your left leg back two feet while pressing your palm against it.
- With your heel still down, bend your right knee slightly while leaning forward until a stretch appears in your left hamstring.
- Hold one or two breaths before releasing, and repeat on the other side.

STANDING KNEE RAISE

- Start standing beside a wall with one hand resting against it as support. Brace your core as you raise your right knee towards your chest.
- As you lift your knee, press your lower back against the wall with pressure as your hip flexes upwards.
- Hold one or two breaths before releasing, and repeat on the other side.

WALL DUMBBELL ARM RAISE

- Start standing against a wall holding two light dumbbells with your elbows bent at 90 degrees in each hand and lift each arm until they reach their maximum potential.

- To perform Brace and Raise Arm Circles, brace your core and slowly raise both arms until they parallel the floor.
- Hold one to two breaths before returning your arms to their original starting positions.

WALLS DB ARM CIRCLES

- To perform Walls DB Arm Circles, stand against a wall while holding two light dumbbells bent at 90-degree angles in your hands and arms outstretched to either side - make sure that both dumbbells have handles!
- Brace your core and raise your arms until they parallel the floor.
- From here, draw small circles in the air for 30 seconds in one direction before switching directions and continuing for another 30 seconds - these exercises are great chest openers!
- Begin by standing against a wall with feet about two feet away, palms flat against it at shoulder height, then bracing your core, pressing your chest against it, and sliding your hands up until your arms have fully extended overhead.

WALL SITS

- Start by standing with your back against a wall, feet about two feet apart, and back against your back until your thighs parallel the floor.
- Gradually slide down the wall until your thighs reach a parallel position before slowly returning up again to the starting position.
- Hold this position for 30 seconds or as long as possible.

SEATED OPPOSITE TOE TAP

- Sit comfortably on the floor with your back against a wall and legs out in front.
- Spread them apart so they are about hip-width apart.
- Stay your core by pressing your lower back into the wall as you perform this exercise.
- Do this exercise by tapping your right toe with your left hand.
- Substitute sides for 45 seconds or as long as possible before switching sides again.

SEATED SPINE TWIST

- Begin this move seated on the floor with your back against a wall and legs straight out in front.
- Attempt a twist using both hands at once by lifting one leg at a time towards you while twisting both arms forward over each shoulder, starting by raising one knee while keeping them apart until your upper body reaches 90 degrees.
- Spread your legs about hip-width apart. Brace your core.
- From here, twist to the right and reach your left hand towards your right leg until it touches the ground outside; reverse this motion by reaching the opposite way for your left leg instead.
- Eventually, reverse your twist by reaching your right hand toward your left leg!
- Substitute sides for 45 seconds or as long as possible,

BUTTERFLY STRETCH.

- On the ground, with the back against the wall and legs bent forward, the soles of your feet touching.
- Let your knees fall to the sides as you press your lower back against the wall.
- Reach your arms above your head and arch your back away from the wall.
- Hold for two breaths, then release back into the starting position.

SEATED FORWARD FOLD

To perform a Seated Forward Fold:

- Sit with your back against a wall while having your legs bent forward, touching the soles of your feet on the ground in front of you with soles touching.
- Let your knees drop to the sides while pressing your lower back against a wall.
- Reach your arms above your head and fold forward from your hips as far as possible while letting your head and shoulders hang weightily on either side.
- Hold for one or two breaths before returning to the starting position.

WEEK 4: MASTERING WALL PILATES FLOW

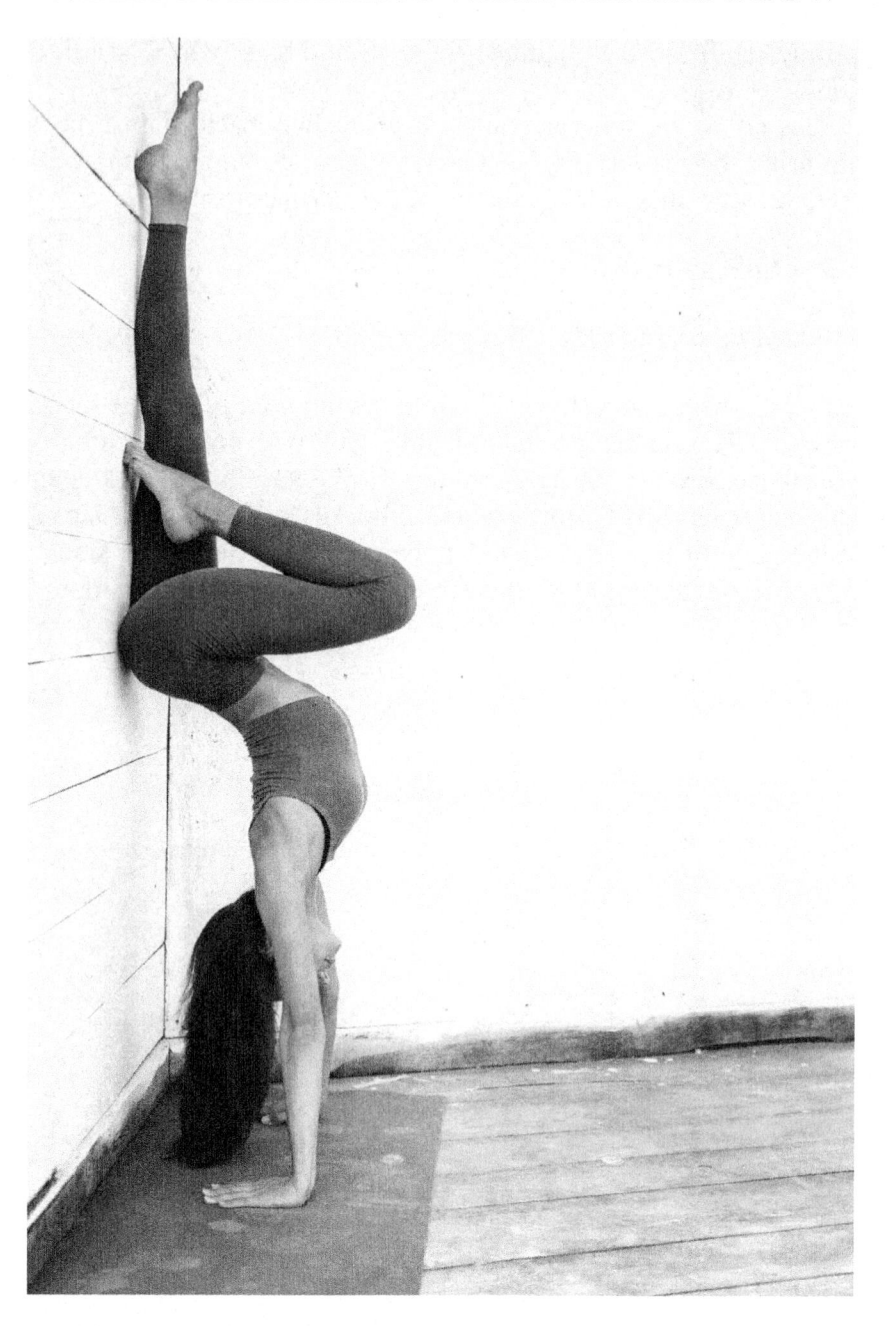

Pilates has a long history of being praised for its profound effects on general well-being and physical conditioning. Numerous people have benefited from its core-strengthening and flexibility-enhancing activities in reaching their fitness and health objectives. But Wall Pilates is a brand-new aspect of Pilates that's blowing up the fitness scene. This creative method uses a wall — you guessed it — to provide a distinctive spin to the classic Pilates technique.

DYNAMIC WALL PILATES ROUTINE

Pilates on a wall combines the support and resistance of the wall with the dynamic approach to training that uses the concepts of Pilates. Anyone who wants to get more flexible, strengthen their core, and improve their overall fitness should consider this. Whatever your degree of familiarity with the discipline, pilates exercises at home.

It offers a fun method to enhance your workout routine and accomplish your health goals.

Wall Pilates might be the full-body exercise you've been looking for. Pilates wall workouts share many characteristics with general Pilates but add unique movements that work your muscles differently.

BREATHING AND CORE ACTIVATION

Before you begin each move, you must activate your core and focus on breathing. You can do this by lying on your back with your knees bent and feet on the floor. Place your hands on your abdomen and inhale through your nose, allowing your hands to slide apart as you breathe into your abdomen. As you exhale, feel your hands slide towards each other, pull your belly button back towards your spine, and engage and lift your pelvic floor. You are now ready to begin!

THE WORKOUT

- Roll down x 5 reps
- Dynamic plank x5 reps per leg
- Superman x5 reps per side
- Side-lying clam shells x10 reps per leg
- Tabletop toe taps x8-10 reps per leg
- The swan x 5-10 reps
- The hundred 1 set of 100 reps
- Roll like a ball x10 reps

A breakdown of each of these moves can be found below.

ROLL DOWN (5 REPS)

We always like to start our classes with a roll down to help mobilize the spine and activate many core muscles, such as the glutes and abs.

Start with your feet hip-width apart and raise your arms above your head as inhale. As you exhale, roll down, keeping your knees soft and maintaining your core, then use your abs and glutes to help bring you back to standing again, finishing by bringing your shoulder blades back and down towards your bottom. Repeat five times.

DYNAMIC PLANK (5 REPS ON EACH LEG)

This move builds that core strength, strengthens your wrists and glutes, and stretches your hamstrings and calves down the backs of your legs.

You start in a plank position before bringing your left knee to your elbow, pushing through your arms, and keeping your core engaged.

You must then activate your shoulders and glutes to push back and kick into a three-legged dog position. Repeat this five times on your left leg before you switch legs, and do five on your right leg.

SUPERMAN (5 REPS ON EACH SIDE)

A core move for any home Pilates workout, the Superman targets the lower and upper body and the care.

Start on all fours on your exercise mat, ensuring that your wrists align with your shoulders and knees in line with your hips. Extend your right leg straight behind you while extending your left arm forward in front of you. Bring the extended arm and leg back to the starting position before repeating with the other arm and leg. Do this ten times, five times per side.

Maintaining good posture and keeping your pelvis neutral (hips in line) through this move is crucial for your balance.

SIDE-LYING CLAM SHELLS (10 REPS PER LEG)

The next exercise in our Pilates routine focuses on core and glute activation and can make you feel the burn!

Lying on your side on your mat with your arm outstretched under your head, bring your legs one on top of the other, your hips stacked. Suck your belly button back towards your spine and engage your pelvic floor to activate your core, then squeeze through your glutes to take your knees apart, then slowly back together. Repeat this ten times per leg.

TABLETOP TOE TAPS (10 REPS)

Lying on your back engages your core and ensures your lower back has good contact with the floor. Lift your legs so your knees align with your hips and your feet are off the floor. Tap alternate toes to the floor, ensuring you maintain good abdominal engagement.

Repeat this 5-10 times per leg; if you lose your core engagement or feel your lower back lifting from the mat, stop and re-engage before continuing.

THE SWAN (5-10 REPS)

This Pilates exercise is a variation on a dorsal raise that targets and strengthens the back muscles but is a great full-body exercise. Be sure to focus on your form for this one.

Start by lying face down on your mat, and engage through your lower back and glutes to lift your chest off the floor. Have your arms extended by your ears before squeezing your elbows back in line with your shoulder blades. Repeat 5-10 times.

THE HUNDRED (1 SET OF 100)

The Hundred is a core Pilates exercise that is great for warming up the core and the shoulders.

Lying on your back, lift your knees and feet off the floor, crunch up, lift your head and upper back off the floor, and engage your core. Extend your legs to where the ceiling and wall meet before you, and extend your arms, keeping them off the floor.

Move your arms up and down as you take five short breaths in and five short breaths out, aiming to beat your arms 100 times. Avoid straining your neck by maintaining good form; bring your legs to the tabletop if you require an easier modification.

ROLL LIKE A BALL (5-10 REPS)

This is a great move to finish a workout as it stretches your back while working those core muscles.

In a seated position, hug your knees into your chest, holding on to your shins. Round through the spine, tucking your chin to your chest, draw your shoulders down, and engage your core.

Roll backward onto your back and shoulders as you inhale, lifting your bottom off the mat. As you exhale, engage the core and roll back to the starting position, keeping your feet off the mat if you want to add more challenge and balance. Repeat ten times.

INCORPORATING PROPS FOR INTENSITY

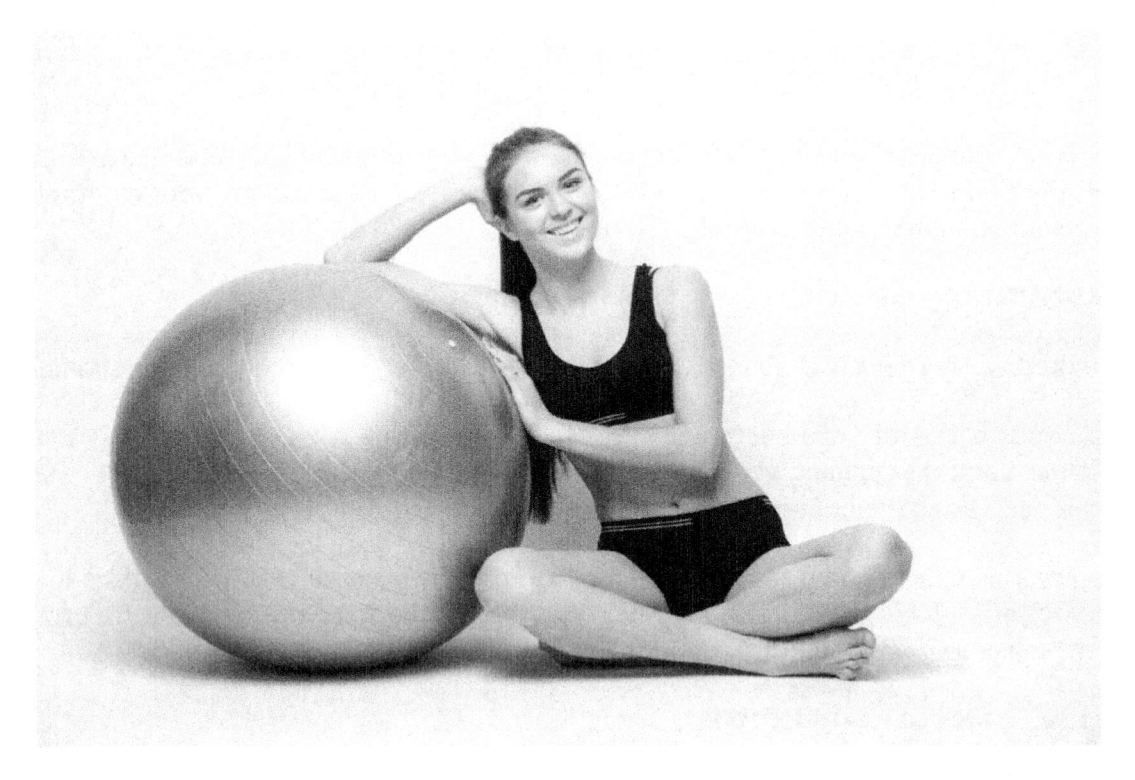

You could utilize props with almost any exercise, but each has a unique feel and setup to accompany them.

BALL

The most adaptable prop we adore is the 10" inch-fit ball. It can provide stability and vigor. It can be put beneath the feet (in poised or bridge position) to test equilibrium; beneath the waist or behind one's back to provide extra assistance in an abdominal sequence; among the your palms or beneath the assisting hand in plank work to improve the concentration on the chest; or in a position among the thighs and ankles for bigger the inner-thigh link; behind the knees for additional hamstring function.

LOOP BAND

The loop band is one of our other favorites. The loop band can be placed over the ankles and knees to intensify the outermost thighs and the abductors, over the foot arches to provide more resistance when working the hamstrings and glutes, or over the wrists and elbows to substitute hand weights. It may assist with stretch as well. The good thing about the loop band is that it comes in a variety of resistances, from extremely light to exceptionally massive, so you can always make a fresh class.

LIGHTWEIGHTS

Lightweights are last, but certainly not least. Since we are able to utilize light weights on our hands for long span of timing and in varied ways to target our muscles in our upper bodies, we adore them. Hand weights are not just good for the hands; they may be utilized in a chair between the legs, right above the knees, or just behind the knee to increase the extent of glute work. Additionally, it may be used in the hands to combine the upper-body activity with the lower body or among both legs for leg lifts and lowers during abdominal exercises. We define lightweights as from one to three pounds and heavyweights as four to five pounds.

You're undoubtedly acquainted with accessories like small balls, balls (Bosu), foam rollers, magic circles, and barres if you have taken a Pilates Matwork with Props class.

BENEFITS OF PILATES PROPS

1. BRINGS AWARENESS TO PROPER ALIGNMENT DURING MOVEMENT

Introducing props helps the body better respond to the tactile feedback the tool provides. Using a circle of magic between your thighs located above the level of your knees to perform upright squats and pelvic twists is a manner of demonstration using a prop for this kind of exercise.

The Magic Circle aligns the knees properly for these exercises as the inner thighs actively squeeze on the pilates ring. The resistance also encourages body weight to be distributed evenly to the balls and heels, bringing the feet and legs into better alignment.

2. ACTIVATES DORMANT MUSCLES

A number of us have lives where we devote most of our days sitting behind a desk for prolonged periods. Props can assist ensure you are using the correct muscles instead of supplementing with the usage of others, particularly for individuals like you to whomever this is applicable. This can lead some muscles into growing weaker or unresponsive.

To guarantee that the core muscles contract, it can be helpful to first relax the front of the chest by placing a small ball beneath one's upper back in chest lifts.

3. ASSISTS AND TRAINS YOU TO DO MOVEMENTS MORE EFFECTIVELY

Some pilates moves can be challenging or too taxing, particularly for individuals who haven't yet built up strength in certain regions of your body.

Props are great to incorporate into a network program to facilitate the execution of these difficult exercises and be sure that they are performed effectively and safely as strength is built over time.

For example, those who lack the abdominal strength to maintain a comfortably lifted head throughout the hundred exercises can prop a Pilates mini ball beneath their upper back.It aids with the motion by raising the head's initial position, avoiding neck strain, and training your body to pivot via the chest rather than the neck.

SUPPORTS CHANGE FOR A HARDER WORKOUT

Even though props could assist you in easing certain exercises, they can also be used to spice up your regular routines and make movements more challenging.

With props, you can manipulate certain movements impacting factors such as variety, unpredictability, and imbalance - all of which help the body perform better and accelerate results in strength, mobility, and flexibility.

Consider a movement such as a Pilates push-up, for example.

Introducing a Bosu ball requires more stability, stepping up the exercise's severity and further encouraging core stability throughout the movement.

COOL DOWN AND STRETCHING ON THE WALL

This is an ideal wall Pilates exercise that works on full-body flexibility as a warm-up and cool-down. In order to get you into the activity portion, it also slightly raises your heart rate.

DIRECTIONS

- Start by firmly planting your complete body on the wall, head to the tailbone included.
- Stretch your feet 6 to 10 inches ahead, contingent on your how tall you are and the shape of your body.
- To lengthen your spine, lift both hands upward until the backs of them contact the wall. Next, start peeling off as you roll each vertebrae individually. Assume that the velcro covering your spine is being peeled away till the toes are exposed.
- When you gain strength, include a walk-out inchworm into this wall Pilates exercise to provide variation. Step forward till the tips of your fingers touch the ground and form a plank-like stance.
- To perform a lunge stretch, put one foot up in ahead of the palm. Do this again on your other side.
- Go back to your plank position and rise up again, experiencing your core tighten as you do so.

CHAPTER 6

MINDFULNESS AND BREATHING METHOD FOR WALL PILATES.

Pilates is an effective exercise method centered on controlled isometric movements and an intricate breathing technique known as the Pilates Breathing Method (PBM). Proper breathing technique is an essential principle in Pilates practice and must be practiced to optimize results from practice sessions.

Pilates uses a technique called posterior-lateral respiration to enhance cardiovascular circulation, promote relaxation, and ease or encourage motion throughout workouts. Three aspects of movement—forward and backwards motion, sideways movement, and three-dimensional movement—are involved in posterior-lateral breathing.

Contrary to diverse types of exercise, posterior-lateral breathing doesn't usually require you to inhale and exhale in response to certain movements - an example that is popularly used in yoga practices as an example is "cat and cow," where you inhale as you arch your back (in the "cow") position and exhale when arching it back up again ("cat" position). Instead, posterior-lateral breathing teaches how to breathe optimally by properly positioning the ribcage.

Are Pilates breathing and Yoga breathing similar?

In yoga, your breath tends to follow the rhythm of your movement; you manage it and coordinate inhales and exhales with different elements of an asana (pose), emphasizing deep abdominal breathing.

BENEFITS OF PROPER BREATHING

As you slowly roll down the spine vertebra by vertebra, notice how your back muscles lengthen. When reaching underneath the roll, exhale as your arms remain parallel to each side.

Breathing correctly during Pilates exercises is critical to achieving maximum results from each routine. Without correct breathing techniques, muscles may fail to engage fully. Furthermore, holding your breath or misusing breathing patterns could prevent reaching the complete motion's range, then reaching your potential.

Benefits of proper breathing may also include:

- Promoting correct muscle activation
- Maintaining abdominal muscle activation
- Preventing shallow breathing.

WHAT ARE THE HEALTH BENEFITS OF PILATES DEEP BREATHING?

Deep breathing through diaphragmatic breathing is one element of Pilates training that may offer you numerous health and well-being advantages.

Physical health benefits may include:

Reducing Stress and Anxiety: Deep breathing and physical exercise can reduce both by increasing your brain's endorphin production and decreasing cortisol. Positive activities that redirect energy away from stressful thoughts can also help alleviate its physical impacts.

Reducing Muscle Tension: Deep breathing helps relax and activate muscles to avoid muscle tension or strain.

Increased Blood Oxygenation: Deep breathing exercises such as those found in Pilates provide additional blood oxygenation to increase energy and productivity throughout your day, providing significant mental health benefits that often surpass physical ones, including:

Keeping emotions balanced: When you breath accurately, it controls the release of feel-good neurotransmitters called dopaminergic and serotonin, relieving stress and creating an atmosphere of tranquility after exercising.

Enhancing Concentration: Exhaling deeply promotes oxygenation and flow to bring blood directly to the brain for easier focus.

Increase Motivation: Exercising and deep breathing together leave you feeling relaxed yet energetic to take on other tasks throughout your day.

DIRECTIONS FOR DOING PILATES BREATHING

Properly doing Pilates breathing, involves inhaling via the nose and breath out via your mouth. Start practicing Pilates breathing without adding additional exercise movements as soon as possible. This should help to establish the foundations of Pilates breathing practice.

While breathing, concentrate on positioning your rib cage in the correct way. When lying flat on a floor or reformers machine, the rib cage ought to appear like it were lying on the flooring and is brought towards the your hips rather than protruding outwards. Your ribs ought not to extend outwardly in this way.

To begin, find the appropriate neutral position:

- Either sit or lie comfortably on the back while bending your legs.
- One hand can be placed on your belly while the other feels your ribs. Keep shoulders unwind and off of your ears.
- Set your spine in an equitable position.
- After you're in position, start breathing techniques using the correct Pilates respiratory sequence.

To correctly apply these:
- Breathe softly via the nostrils as you fill your torso with oxygen and stretch your rib cage.
- To start, gradually raise your abdomen to meet the spine by contracting your transversal abdomen muscles, then releasing your stomach.
- Inhale via the mouth in the absence of air being forced out, without forcing air out at all costs.
- Do this breathing activity several times, focusing on expanding the ribs' front, back, and sideways.

Once you've learned basic breathing techniques, gradually incorporate them into your Pilates workouts to do exercises with appropriate form. To stay a part of the feeling and be able to complete every task correctly, slowly integrate appropriate respiration into your daily life.

Pilates can enhance durability, adaptability, and versatility in motion while assisting with mental and physical equilibrium. Philosophy provides one-on-one coaching, explosive jumpboard classes, and Pilates reformer courses. Find your fitness journey at Philosophy!

BONUS CHAPTER

FITNESS PLANNER FOR SUCCESS

It's simple to start a wall-based Pilates practice; maintaining it takes effort. If you've followed this instructions, you should be well-equipped to begin your training and select the best class to continue with diversity and friendship as you develop together.

Maintain a positive outlook. Recall that all physical activity is a practice, and that there are only infinitely lovely variants rather than perfection.

Practice self-compassion and pay attention to your body. When you find it difficult to maintain your habit or lack motivation, start small and keep yourself responsible to that minimal. Try practicing Pilates wall movements for five minutes, as an example. Permit yourself to quit if it becomes too difficult to go on (but you may discover that you can persevere over the first mental obstacle).

Bear in mind that certain wall Pilates exercises may seem strange or difficult at first, so be open to new experiences. Keeping an open mind can aid you to remain upbeat and confident. Because you're concentrated on mastering every step, it will also aid in keeping you safe.

Each everyone learns new habits differently and it takes different amounts of time for them to completely integrate into their lives. But the great thing about Pilates routines on the wall is that it allows you to practice them whenever and wherever you have free time.

With a little perseverance and patience, you'll soon experience physical and mental well-being gains, and a fun new activity you can do with the people you care about: wall Pilates.

SETTING REALISTIC WALL PILATES GOALS

Embarking on any health and wellness challenge is exciting, but initially, feeling daunting is normal. It's critical to enter the event knowing precisely what you hope to accomplish in order to make the best of it. Indeed, one of the greatest things about fitness is that everyone has distinct objectives. If you've decided to embark on the Amplify Competition, here are five ideas to assist you keep yourself responsible.

The simplest method to divide things down is into SMART goals.

SPECIFIC: Describe your intentions in detail

Focus on specifics rather than a broad objective like "I desire to get active." What specific goals do you currently have in mind? For instance, "I hope to be capable of doing the entire footwork series on six springs" or "I want to maintain Hundreds Level 2 for the whole exercise".

MEASURABLE: QUANTIFY YOUR PROGRESS

Quantify your goals to track progress. Setting a goal like this might help you achieve strength: "I am going to utilize more springs in the footwork series from 4 to 5 by the conclusion of your challenge." If flexibility is your target, you might aim to attend 1 Stretch Class every week for the length of the task.

ACHIEVABLE: Maintain realism

Although it is admirable to push oneself and aim high, ensure your objectives are realistic in light of your existing degree of fitness, your schedule, and additional obligations. It appears more realistic to begin with the goal of attending 4 Pilates classes each week rather than instantly striving for a total of seven classes.

IMPORTANT: MATCH WITH YOUR LARGER PICTURE

Make sure your ambitious life goals align with your Pilates challenge. Include meditation in your workouts if your goal is stress reduction. If losing bodyweight is your goal, adjust how you eat in addition to your Pilates practice.

Temporary: Assign Miles

Even while a six-week period can seem brief, absence of any intermediate goals might make it seem never-ending. Divide your primary objective into smaller, weekly or biweekly objectives. As an illustration, in the first few weeks of mastering a difficult exercise, concentrate on mastering its core postures.

Bonus Advice for Remaining on Course

- Document Your Trip: Make use of your trackers and consult your Boost Health Guide. Observe your lessons, the activities, how you feel both during and afterwards, and any advancements you make.

- Shut your eyes prior to each session and see yourself performing the tasks with ease. This will help you envisage success. A psychological warm-up like this will improve your athletic ability.
- Remain Responsible: Communicate your objectives with a trusted person or collaborate with an acquaintance. During occasions that your personal drive wanes, you may find motivation through this outside scrutiny.
- Honor minor victories: Finished a mini-task? Enjoy a nourishing meal or a therapeutic massage as a manner of marking the occasion.

Setting SMART goals will help you make the best of your subsequent fitness and health quest and can distinguish between an unproductive and effective six-week span. You're setting yourself up for success if you prioritize importance, achievability, measurement capability, precision, and time. Now spread out your mat, make some SMART objectives, and start your change!

USING THE FITNESS PLANNER EFFECTIVELY

A well-structured strategy is the greatest method to achieve your wellness and fitness objectives. If not, all that you're doing is hurling objects at the wall and praying they stay, or whatsoever the expression is.

But for that reason, it's crucial to build up a workout planner!

I understand that creating a weekly workout schedule can be difficult. I have experienced that. I have been so consumed by the idea that I haven't even tried to create a functional exercise planner.

You could try out many things, but to help you out, I compiled seven tips for creating a fitness planner with what I've learned so far on my planning journey.

Let's reach our goals this year!

USE YOUR PLANNER TO CREATE A PLAN

A fitness workout planner needs a plan. As fitness instructors or run coaches have no doubt told you, to see results, it's necessary to create and stick to an actionable plan - this statement holds!

Movement of any sort is always better than inactivity. However, if you aim to build muscle, increase endurance or flexibility, or something else, planning your fitness route should not be random but targeted toward what suits you best. So before buying the first fitness planner you find, ask yourself these important questions:

- How will I structure my workouts? (i.e., the particular workout you will engage in and the days you will engage in it)
- Which metrics am I interested in tracking in my planner (miles traveled, push-up records? Whatever metrics matter to you)?
- Do I prioritize daily, weekly, or monthly tracking, and which pages am I required?

Similarly, research first if you prefer making your plan without an instructor or coach's assistance. Know your fitness goals and learn the techniques used to reach them; this is safer and will ensure a plan that brings results!

Fitness planners won't work unless you invested the work themselves. Make a plan prior to creating your fitness planner to make it even more effective.

1. SELECT AN APPROPRIATE FITNESS PLANNER

When you look for a plan for your fitness, and planner, numerous people and brands will offer advice about a more effective method to plan.

But the reality is that the perfect fitness planner won't necessarily work for EVERYONE. Our minds work differently; we have unique motivators, organizational abilities, and organizational strategies.

Your friend's fitness planner template could be the perfect match that you could work with, too - or it might not.

As a professional runner, I tried many fitness planners over time. If a cute one caught my eye at a store, I'd grab it immediately; watching what other elite runners did and trying to replicate it were always futile attempts that eventually failed (usually rapidly).

As soon as I accepted that everyone has different planning needs than me - and accepted this fact - was when I finally stuck to a plan that worked for me. If that is the case for you, check your workout planner to ensure enough space for fitness meal planning unless this works for you, too.

As a DIY planner, I enjoy putting everything together myself. Pre-made planners don't suit me; fitness planner printables and then "develop yours" planners have become my go-to options ever since I discovered them.

2. TAKE TIME TO UNDERSTAND WHY YOU REQUIRE A FITNESS PLANNER

No one likes doing something without an end in sight. Even if something doesn't appear pointless at first glance, knowing its true purpose remains key in realizing its potential impact on daily life.

Track and field has taught me an invaluable lesson about motivation. When a coach gives challenging workouts without explaining why, it becomes much harder for athletes to feel motivated to give it their all.

By understanding why certain workouts or running drills will benefit your performance, gaining motivation to complete them effectively can give these exercises their intended effect and serve as motivation for doing them well. Utilizing fitness planners provides similar benefits.

3. DON'T FORGET TO SET GOALS

A good piece fitness advice I have received was setting goals - yet due to being intimidated by them; I ignored this advice for too long - big mistake!

Setting goals isn't about being the best in the world or reaching high performance, although that can include some sort of it. Instead, goal setting serves as motivation and inspiration on a journey and provides tangible results where otherwise there would only be aspiration.

Novice runners may choose to register for a 5k six months to a year out as their starting point. Even if you don't intend to win or beat everyone in your community (though this can also be beneficial), creating an end goal provides motivation. It gives a sense of direction when training backward.

You will naturally want to prepare as soon as a race is scheduled. Knowing there will be something on the horizon can serve as motivation, whether running without stopping for any walking breaks or bettering a time you set previously.

To improve your chances of making improvement, set clear objectives and record them in your exercise planner. I suggest dedicating an entire page of your planner for goals or adding specific goals on an events calendar to monitor your development towards specific targets.

4. IMPLEMENT A HABIT TRACKER

Big-picture goals are great, but they will become too lofty and impossible for you without breaking them down into more manageable steps.

I like to work backward from goals. If X is my primary goal, what smaller steps must occur for it to come true? And which daily tangible steps should I take for these smaller goals? Below are two quick examples; for more on habit trackers and why they're great tools, I discuss that further in my post on building healthy habits.

Goal: Run a mile in 5:35.

Lesser Goal One: Increase my long run distance up to six miles

- Lesser Goal Two: is to run a mile-paced workout (this could be more specific, but for this example, we're keeping it easy)
- Lesser Goal Three: Squat 150 pounds for three reps (it's unnecessary if you treat this goal extremely seriously. as an example. For now).

Habits to reach those goals:

- Protein shake after every hard workout
- Eight hours of restful sleep each night.
- Roll Out Sessions 4 Times Weekly

Do you understand where I'm heading here? Keeping a habit tracker can be a good method of gradually adjust to anything difficult for you, as well as helping you reach bigger goals more quickly.

Start small when setting goals and habits while creating your planner - it might seem time-consuming at first, but I promise it works!

5. ALLOCATE AN AREA IN YOUR FITNESS PLANNER FOR EMOTIONAL NOTES

Don't Be Afraid of Your Feelings!

For years, I tried hard to keep my emotions in check as everyone around me made it seem like I should always remain positive. Even within sports, there's often talk of only having positive attitudes, putting down one's head, and grinding.

Though most people had good intentions when they said this to me as a young, impressionable athlete, all I heard was, "Hide your true emotions and pretend everything is just fine always."

Also, that had a lasting effect. Out of fear of sounding negative, I often kept my feelings to myself or used superficial grievances as an outlet. At some point during that period, I realized the value of journaling about emotions.

Do not suppress your emotions on any fitness journey, as there will inevitably be difficult days that require special consideration and recognition. Be prepared for them!

All this is to say that leaving space in your fitness planner for emotions is important. Please don't feel obliged to write an essay about them; note how that workout affected you, whether extra tiredness had set in, sore spots on your body, etc.

This information is essential to your fitness, allowing you to tailor your training load. If you're having a bad day, switch out a hard workout for something lighter, or if a type of activity makes your legs sore afterward, be mindful not to schedule another hard, long sprint day directly afterward.

Many journals enable recording your feelings as easy as jotting down an optimistic or pessimistic face on each day's page. Take the time to record any information or feelings you want in an attempt to build an effective fitness planner.

6. MAKE YOUR FITNESS PLANNER AESTHETICALLY PLEASING

Although some might scoff at this idea, it should look nice if something needs to be looked at daily. There's no excuse not to put some effort into creating your workout schedule. Look appealing while simultaneously getting down to business!

No matter what floats your boat, make it work for you! Aim for something that inspires rather than becomes another monotonous task.

As previously discussed in an earlier tip, finding the ideal planner can make all the difference in sticking with a fitness planner. I spoke specifically about setting up the fitness planner template and its aesthetic qualities.

So how can one make the best workout planner?

- Utilize inspirational quote cards or write directly on pages for motivation. It put motivational dashboards throughout the pages. And use fitness planner stickers.
- These small adjustments can make your workout scheduler a factor you look forward to using and will be happy to utilize.
- You could get greater results with a computerized fitness planner, with plenty of customization options for creating stunning digital fitness planners.

Time To Get Planning!

Obviously, setting yourself up for fitness planner success requires many strategies; I hope these seven tips have given you some ideas of where to begin. They are straightforward concepts you can easily put into action: get yourself an attractive planner with goals set and track why they matter.

My most efficient fitness planner is just a note on my iPhone app! It works beautifully to meet my goals quickly.

However, a more robust plan may become necessary as my life changes and my routine evolves. Remember this: whenever you feel overwhelmed by setting up a fitness planner - it may look different at different times! And that's okay - each phase in our life requires something unique!!

NUTRITION TIPS FOR WALL PILATES SUCCESS

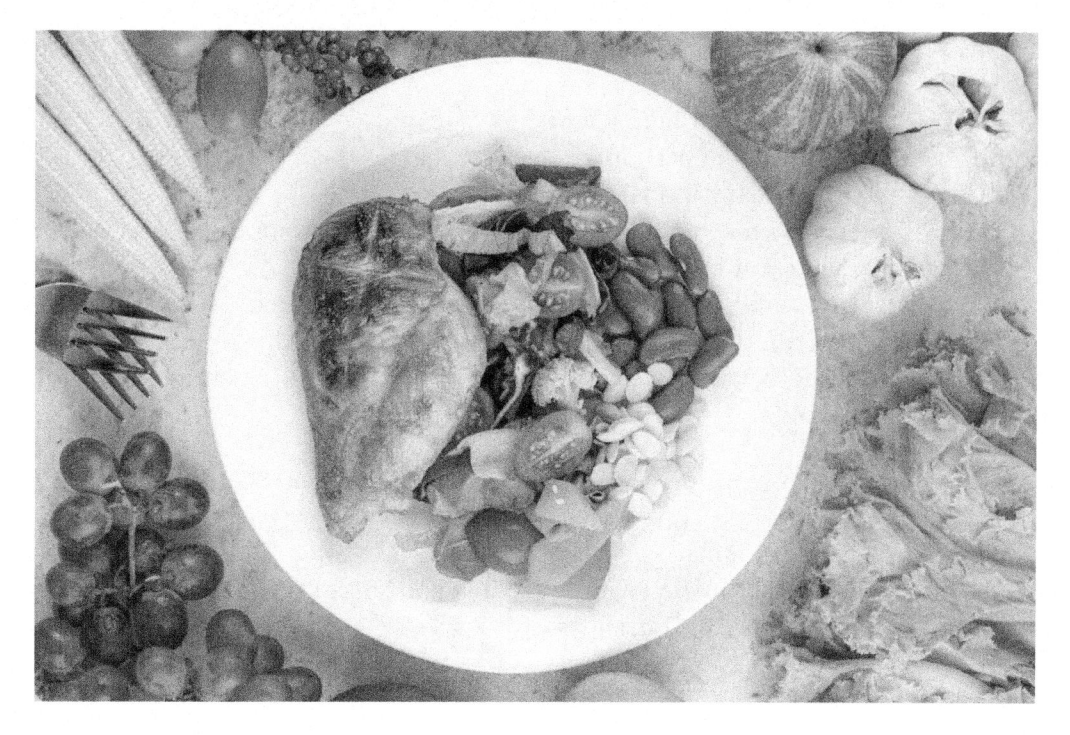

Wellness Pilates workouts offer a variety of advantages, like enhanced flexibility, toned muscles from head to toe, better balance, and improved mobility. Enhancing your body's nutritional intake might augment the advantages of Pilates.

We've compiled a complete guide on your diet while practicing Pilates, such as whatever to eat, and the time to consume it prior to and following a Pilates session, the importance of staying hydrated during workouts, and pre and post-workout snack and meal ideas.

WHEN TO EAT BEFORE PILATES CLASS

Not only the food you eat before a workout matters, but also when you consume it. It is not advisable to have a big meal that hasn't fully digested before going to class. Believe us, following a large dinner, hundreds are not enjoyable!

While everyone is different when it comes to the ideal time to eat before working exercise, there are some basic rules to go by. Try not to eat anything an hour before your lesson. You could even choose to give yourself two hours to go between meals and your Pilates session.

Try varying the timing and food combinations to see what suits you the best.

If you eat too little just before a Pilates lesson, you could experience dizziness or fatigue. You may feel sluggish and uncomfortable after eating too much.

- Before choosing what to consume just before a Pilates session, bear the following advice in mind:
- Stay away from foods that cause gas or bloating (i.e., cabbage, onions, lentils, beans, cauliflower, broccoli, and garlic)
- Avoid foods that are heavy or take a while to digest
- Steer clear of foods heavy in carbohydrates or sugar.
- Avoid large meals or greasy foods
- Avoid foods high in sugar and carbs, as they elevate your blood sugar concentrations as well as crash, leaving you low energy.
- Rather, concentrate upon a small supper or eat a snack that contains complex carbohydrates, protein that is lean, and nutritious fats. This mixture can assist you maintain appropriate levels of energy while keeping you energized so you can go throughout the lesson.

• Choose a light option, like as a tiny bowl of yogurt covered with berries plus almonds or a banana drizzled with nut butter, for your early-morning Pilates workouts.

• An energy-dense meal, like an omelet with avocados and salsa on top, will offer a healthy full energy level for your afternoon Pilates lessons.

Below are some healthy pre-workout snacks and meals you should eat an hour or two before attending your Pilates class:

- Scrambled eggs with avocado and some fresh berries on top
- Unsweetened yogurt topped with fruit and nuts
- An apple with nut butter and a tiny cheese cube.
- A side dish of lush dark greens with chopped hard-boiled egg and almonds on top;
- A wrap made of lettuce featuring lean proteins such as turkey;
- A banana using almond spread
- The combination of celery with hummus
- Create a green smoothie using leafy greens, half a banana, berries, and unsweetened plain yogurt;
- Select a protein bar that is unsweetened and free of preservatives and extra sweeteners.
- An excellent protein shake (once more, be sure to read the contents carefully)
- A tiny cup of oats with a few strawberries on top
- Nut spread with a few baby carrots or strawberries on whole grain toast that has sprouted.

Additionally, it is suggested for you to avoid consuming a lot of carbohydrates prior to session.

EATING TIMES AFTER PILATES CLASSES

It's crucial to eat a modest meal or snack between thirty and sixty minutes following your Pilates session. This gives your body the lean protein it requires in order to rebuild your muscles and replenishes the glycogen stores in your body.

THINGS TO EAT AFTER THE PILATES SESSION

You should consume complex carbohydrates, lean proteins, and healthy fats, after the activity.

These are a few quick and wholesome post-Pilates dinner suggestions:

- A tasty and simple post-workout snack is a protein smoothie prepared with premium protein powder and nutritious components.
- One bowl of plain Greek yogurt with fruit and nuts on top and an accompanying boiled egg are also healthy choices.
- For an easy lunch option that's full of veggies, try this veggie-packed omelet featuring spinach, asparagus, onion, mushrooms, bell peppers, black olives, and diced avocado (the last ingredient can also be swapped out if desired):
- Sweet potato with fish or grilled chicken
- Grilled chicken served over brown rice alongside non-starchy vegetables
- Create a delicious salad featuring diced boiled egg, pistachios, bell pepper, sunflower seeds, and your other favorite veggies as toppings.

For optimal recovery post-class, ensure your body receives an assortment of fats, proteins, and carbohydrates.

What to Eat During the Pilates Routines

The objectives and your physique will influence how you ought to nourish yourself between your Pilates sessions, however consuming in proportion will assist you develop strong, lean muscles and maintain a steady level of energy to guarantee that you're ready at all times for the following session.

Aim to eat a diet high in complete, foods that are rich in nutrients, such as seeds, nuts, and nut butter; nuts from wild-caught sources (sardines, salmon, tuna, or anchovies); unsweetened yogurt; fruits; vegetables and leafy greens

Healthy living requires choosing whole grains for breakfast, such as quinoa, millet, brown rice, wheat, or outdated oatmeal.

Every nutritious eating routine should center around lean protein, which may be found in chicken, turkey, fish, eggs, and full-fat dairy products. Maintaining balance while dieting is important to achieve lasting success; don't restrict yourself too severely by including high-quality desserts now and again, making it a portion of a long-term success strategy.

BENEFITS OF STAYING HYDRATED

As you sweat, fluid is lost from your body. To replenish these losses and maximize performance during workouts, adequate hydration must be maintained by drinking enough fluids during each session. Without sufficient fluid intake during a workout session, fatigue increases substantially, as does impaired thinking abilities, bodily processes as well as diminished effectiveness in sports.

During exercise, drinking enough of water has several benefits, such as:

- Sustain bodily functions along with performance standards
- Reduce the likelihood of stress caused by heat
- Aid in preventing a rise in body temperature or heartbeat
- Increase endurance
- Enhance concentration
- Keep the blood volume constant.

- Boost your level of energy and assist the body's normal detoxification processes.

- Boost Your Metabolic Rate

Thirty minutes before your Pilates session, have a minimum of an eight-ounce glass of water to be hydrated. Keep a water bottle nearby during class so you can sip as needed.

CONCLUSION

Although it's always in trend, Pilates is currently seeing a major upsurge in recognition. The fact that Pilates is so widely available serves as a good purpose for its popularity. Very little equipment is needed to adapt routines to each person's needs, preferences, and restrictions. A yoga mat plus a wall are needed to accomplish this wall Pilates exercise. It receives no less upkeep than that.

However, while doing a Pilates exercise on the wall doesn't involve a lot of sophisticated equipment, you shouldn't write it off as simple. Pilates on a wall constitutes an amazing full-body, low-impact workout suitable for several stages of activeness to promote control, steadiness, power, and posture.

One option of the numerous methods for simulating reformer Pilates at home is wall Pilates, using the wall to imitate its resistance to bring reformer-like activities to your schedule. Elevating your feet during this workout may increase circulation, digestion, and sleep quality, also to minimize muscle cramps, not to mention its many other benefits! Wall Pilates will add something different and exciting to any mat Pilates workout routine! Just like a kettlebell or a yoga block, a wall is only an instrument. It may be useful for adaptations. After surgery, you might use a wall to perform pushup variants. Additionally, it might be beneficial for exercises that develop the motion's level, such as sit-ups. Plus, it's free.

I recommend performing a single wall Pilates activity during a 30-minute Pilates session.

Do wall Pilates if it's a practice you look forward to, like, and can stick with. Try a different thing if not. Fads are fads, so avoid pushing yourself to follow them just because you've observed someone else on social media doing it. looking all, a workout is a very small piece of the picture if results are what you're looking. Pleasure takes precedence over everything.

Printed in Great Britain
by Amazon